Geriatrics in the United States

**Manpower Projections
and Training Considerations**

D0930541

Robert L. Kane
The Rand Corporation
U.C.L.A. School of Medicine
David H. Solomon
U.C.L.A. School of Medicine
John C. Beck
U.C.L.A. School of Medicine
Emmett B. Keeler
The Rand Corporation
Rosalie A. Kane
The Rand Corporation

LexingtonBooks
D.C. Heath and Company
Lexington, Massachusetts
Toronto

Library of Congress Cataloging in Publication Data

Main entry under title:

Geriatrics in the United States.

Includes bibliographical references and index.
1. Gerontologists—United States—Supply and demand. 2. Geriatrics—Study and teaching—United States. I. Kane, Robert Lewis, 1940–
[DNLM: 1. Geriatrics—Manpower—United States. 2. Training support. WT 21 K16g]
RC952.5.G444   1981   331.12'3161897'00973   80–8840
ISBN 0–669–04386–9

Published simultaneously in Canada

Printed in the United States of America

International Standard Book Number: 0–669–04386–9

Library of Congress Catalog Card Number: 80–8840

Contents

Contents

List of Figures
and Tables

Preface

This study, supported by the Henry J. Kaiser Family Foundation, was designed to provide quantitative estimates of the geriatric manpower that might be required over the next fifty years in the United States. A variety of models have been proposed, based on the recommendations of professional groups. The projections offered are intended only as boundary estimates, serving to put quantitative bounds on what have heretofore been primarily qualitative statements. This report is intended to be used by policymakers, educators, and others interested in the training and deployment of geriatric personnel.

The elderly are a vulnerable group in our society—a group whose numbers are growing. Although they are consumers of extensive medical-care services, these services are generally not tailored to their needs. This book uses demographic and utilization data to project the needs for physician personnel to provide care for the elderly over the next fifty years. The quantitative estimates are then coupled with qualitative analyses to seek better means of delivering the needed services. We conclude that a corps of specially trained individuals is desperately needed; estimates of its size are given later in this preface. Our numerical estimates should be viewed as targets, unattainable by 1990, possibly attainable by 2010 or 2020. It will be difficult enough in the near future to train a sufficient number of geriatricians to serve as faculty for training primary-care providers who will likely continue to offer most of the care to the aged in this country.

Those 65 years of age and older currently number over 23 million (almost 11 percent of the United States population). By the year 2030 this age group will more than double to 55 million (almost 20 percent of the population). The group over age 75 will then be as large as is the over-65 group today.

The aged represent a population at risk. They are often the victims of multiple handicaps—physical, social, and economic. Those who would care for them adequately need the requisite skills to mobilize the variety of resources necessary to respond to this multifocal assault on the aged. A complex mixture of medical and social needs in the midst of inflation keeps the elderly poorly served and often forgotten, in spite of Social Security and Medicare. A few statistics may help to portray the plight of the elderly:

Eighty-five percent of the elderly suffer from at least one chronic condition of ill health.

Fifty-six percent of those over age 75 (and 42 percent of those over age 65) are limited in activity because of chronic conditions.

Those over age 75 have almost twice as many bed-disability days and restricted-activity days as those aged 45 to 64.

The rate of entry into nursing homes is twenty-five times higher among those 75 and over, compared with those 45 to 64.

In fiscal year 1977 the per-capita health expenditure for those aged 65 and over was almost three times that for the 19-to-64 age group ($1,745 compared with $661).

The median income of heads of households over age 65 is less than half that for all household heads.

Thirty-seven percent of elderly women live alone.

In the 1977 Physician Survey conducted by the American Medical Association (AMA), less than 0.6 percent of the respondents indicated an interest in geriatrics.

Physicians spend less time per visit with elderly patients, even though the elderly have more numerous diseases and more complicated social problems.

To provide medical care to the elderly, the geriatrician must have knowledge and skills distinct from those offered by other physicians. Not only is the presentation of disease often different, but its management will vary with the social and economic environment. The geriatrician must be much more of a manager than the ordinary physician, since he must be capable of mobilizing resources and looking at a patient's total environment. He needs a different (or at least an additional) set of measures that address the patient's total functioning and are sufficiently sensitive to identify areas of success, as well as to document the need for further therapy.

Research in geriatrics will examine a variety of areas from biomedical investigations of the basis of aging to analyses of health services that will seek better ways of meeting the health-care needs of the elderly. Particular emphasis should be placed on examining the underlying mechanisms that account for much of the disability and subsequent use of services. These topics include diseases of the joints, incontinence, confusion, falls, and loss of mobility. In addition, the social and environmental factors exacerbating these problems deserve further study.

In this book we have identified four possible levels of geriatric activity as a basis for our estimates of manpower needs:

1. A continuation of the current care-delivery pattern, with essentially no specially trained geriatricians.
2. Geriatricians trained primarily for academic positions, but with some inevitable spillover into practice.

3. Academic geriatricians plus a trained cohort of geriatric consultants, as are found in much of Western Europe.
4. Geriatricians in academic roles and actively involved in practice as both consultants and providers of substantial amounts of primary care.

Recognizing the shortfalls of physician manpower in geriatrics, we have gone on to estimate the effects of sharing the care of elderly patients with nurse practitioners (NPs), physician's assistants (PAs), and social workers (SWs). The resultant model provides for twelve variations (four styles of practice with three levels of delegation for each).

We estimate a need for at least 900 academic geriatricians just to staff existing training programs in internal medicine and family practice, as well as to provide a core group of geriatricians in each medical school. This would mean training at least 1,500 geriatricians to allow for losses.

For practicing geriatricians, the range of estimates is much wider. Today we would require 195 geriatricians to give care to those age 75 and older at the current level (leaving most of the responsibility for the care of the elderly on the shoulders of primary-care physicians and, to a lesser extent, medical specialists); but if we want to have geriatricians rendering some primary care to those aged 65 and older, more than 16,000 would be needed today. This number could be reduced by about a third if maximum use of NPs, PAs, and SWs were made. By the year 2030 there would be a need for only 515 geriatricians to maintain the status quo for those aged 75 and older; but almost 38,000 would be needed to provide academic leadership, consultation, and some primary care for those aged 65 and older. If we include in our estimates some adjustment for improved care, the latter figure increases to more than 47,000.

The authors' point of choice along this spectrum is defined by the following assumptions:

1. Most specialized geriatric care will be directed at persons 75 and older.
2. The academic complement and the geriatric specialist in community settings are essential for the desired quality of care, and a moderate amount of primary care by geriatricians will occur as a not-undesirable byproduct.
3. At least a moderate degree of delegation of care to NPs, PAs, and SWs will be feasible and desirable.
4. We should aim for an increment of improved care for the elderly.

With these assumptions, this country will require between 7,000 and 10,300 geriatricians by 1990, the best intermediate estimate being about 8,000.

These estimates of needed geriatric manpower are based on a proposed redistribution of physician-training efforts rather than on an absolute increase in the number of physicians. When compared with the currently available geriatric training programs, the shortfall is enormous. Suggestions are made in the course of this book for changes in direction. Clearly, a substantial influx of resources will be required to establish the academic milieu necessary to recruit and train the number of geriatricians needed in the future. Although there have been recent signs of growing academic-health-center interest in the production of geriatric manpower, these efforts are inadequate.

This report focuses on the projected activities of physicians and closely related health providers in redressing the inadequate care of the elderly. This emphasis should not be interpreted as insensitivity to the very important role of those who provide nonmedical care or as a failure to consider other models of care, in which physicians play a more technical, less central role. Although there is some cogency to limited physician participation, there are great perils in that approach. The distinction between medical and social models is more artificial than real. More germane is the danger that such a strategy may be attractive for perverse reasons. The physician's indifference to the aged is part of the problem; the solution is not likely to be found in excluding physicians or in allowing them to exclude themselves. Moreover, the history of sociomedical progress strongly argues that physician participation brings to bear power, prestige, and performance. All are surely lacking at present with regard to the aged. A more satisfactory compromise appears to lie in developing physician leaders who can work with other professionals to develop an integrated approach to the care of the elderly.

A series of recommendations is offered in the final chapter of this book. These include:

1. Increasing training programs for health professionals in geriatrics.
2. Strengthening required undergraduate programs in geriatrics.
3. Expanding the teaching of geriatrics in primary-care training programs.
4. Increasing geriatric fellowships.
5. Strengthening geriatric professional societies.
6. Developing visible geriatric units in each medical school.
7. Offering professional recognition for advanced training in geriatrics.
8. Changing payment schemes to reward more personal care.
9. Accrediting geriatric training programs.
10. Increasing the use of geriatric nurse practitioners (GNPs) and PAs in delivering geriatric care.
11. Amending state pharmacy laws to allow GNPs to write prescriptions for certain drugs.
12. Amending Medicare regulations to facilitate payment of GNPs and PAs in geriatric practice without on-site physician supervision.
13. Developing an academic cadre of GNPs.

14. Increasing clinical and health-services research in geriatrics.
15. Developing a better data set on all health professionals in geriatrics.
16. Developing a standardized set of measures and vocabulary with regard to the care of the elderly.

Acknowledgments

Many people provided us with invaluable assistance in gathering data for this project. Robert Mendenhall, director of medical activities and manpower projects, Division of Research in Medical Education, University of Southern California, provided special analyses of his data on physician productivity. Edwin Perrin sent us his report on the validity and reliability of the University of Southern California Physician Manpower Study. Gene Roback and Donald Donais graciously provided a copy of the American Medical Association 1977 Physician Survey data tape. Mary Grace Kovar supplied data on the health status and use of health services by the elderly from the National Center for Health Statistics. Owen Beard and Eugene Towbin graciously sent unpublished data from their Geriatric Evaluation Unit at the Little Rock Veterans Administration Hospital.

John Graettinger, Peter Weil, and Alvin Tarlov provided data on postgraduate education; Peter Dans, information from the Institute of Medicine report on geriatrics; Theodore Reiff, information on geriatric training programs; Thomas Morgan, of the Association of American Colleges, and William Batchelor, of the National Institutes of Health, information on the outcomes of federally supported training programs; and Ralph Goldman and John Mather, data on the geriatric training programs developed by the Veterans Administration.

Our assessment of the state of geropsychiatry was greatly assisted by a panel that included Lissy Jarvik, Manuel Straker, and R. Bruce Sloane. Further data on geropsychiatry was provided by James Birren, Carolyn Robinowitz, and Carl Eisdorfer.

A number of persons advised us on the state of information concerning other health specializations in geriatrics: physical therapy—Rita Ruskin, James Clinkingbeard, Joanne Mills, and Royce Noland; podiatry—Seward Nyman; speech-language-hearing—Kathleen Griffin; nursing—Irene Burnside, Myrtle Aydolott, Doris Schwartz, Sister Erica Bunké, Aleda Roth, Naomi Potchin, and Laurie Gunter; dentistry—William Borman and Ronald Ettinger; social work—Robert Cohen; pharmacy—Lars Solander; occupational therapy—Francis Acquaviva; optometry—Stephen Miller and R. Averill.

During the course of the project, many persons provided useful comments on our formulations. These included John Brocklehurst, Robert Butler, Caroll Estes, A. Norman Exton-Smith; Christopher Foote, Neta Foote, David Kennie, Bernard Isaacs, Philip Lee, Leslie Libow, Michael Lye, George Maddox, Sean McCarthy, Robert Morris, Balfour Mount, K. Warner Schaie, Sylvia Sherwood, T. Franklin Williams, and Elenud Woodford-Williams.

The *Los Angeles Times* kindly allowed us to reprint the material shown in appendix A. Alan Robbins and Itamar Abrass were major contributors to the educational objectives shown in appendixes C and D.

We wish to extend thanks to the reviewers of an earlier draft of this book, whose insightful comments contributed substantially to its final form: Paul Beeson, Alfred Sadler, and Robert Brook. Jonathan Meyer served as research assistant throughout the project and made contributions to the overall report. Finally, we wish to thank Janice Jones, whose diligence and unending patience with seemingly endless revisions of the book were major factors in our completing the task. The authors, of course, assume all responsibility for the final product.

We wish to express our special thanks to Robert Glaser, president of the Henry J. Kaiser Family Foundation, for his continuous support throughout the course of this project.

1 Introduction

Medical educators and policymakers have sounded alarms at the failure of medical education to prepare graduates to meet the needs of a major segment of the population, the elderly. Fears of current inadequacy of care resources are heightened by demographic forecasts that show that the number of elderly, particularly of the very elderly, are growing substantially in both absolute and relative terms. Because the elderly use more services per capita than do younger persons, their relative growth is as important as their absolute growth. This demographic imperative demands a response.

Any call for additional manpower to meet the projected increase in utilization of medical services does not harmonize well with the more somber predictions about the growth of academic medicine. Rogers (1980) foresees the 1980s as a time of substantially restricted funding for research and teaching. New programs will generally have to replace old ones if they are to find support in a no-growth environment. It is indeed a difficult time to give birth to geriatrics, but this country is already more than a little pregnant.

The recent report of the National Academy of Sciences' Institute of Medicine (IOM 1978; Dans and Kerr 1979) recommends that medical-educational programs provide more coverage of geriatrics and related material in gerontology, but it does not suggest the creation of new cadres of practitioners. The responsibility for providing geriatric care would remain vested in the establishment; but newly sensitized, medical specialties of geriatrics and gerontology would be recognized as academic disciplines in the medical school.

The IOM report, combined with statements from the American Geriatrics Society and other groups, impressively documents the contention that geriatric care needs attention. However, some detractors still maintain that care is already being provided by primary-care physicians and specialists (especially in internal medicine) who possess sufficient skill and knowledge to perform the necessary tasks.

This debate about the need for redirection of physician manpower into geriatric care centers around a series of questions to be addressed in this book.

1. Is there a problem with the care currently provided to the elderly?
2. If a problem does exist, might it be solved by redirecting personnel, or are more physicians needed?

1

3. What roles should geriatricians play? Should we plan for academic
    geriatricians only? If practicing geriatricians are required, should they
    follow the specialist model of some nations in Western Europe?
4. Are the knowledge, attitudes, and skills specifically associated with
    geriatrics adequate to designate the field as a separate discipline?

These questions raise yet another set of questions more directly aimed
at issues of training:

5. How much manpower is desirable for the health care of the elderly, as
    well as for teaching and research in geriatrics?
6. Can we identify configurations of geriatric personnel that are effective
    and efficient?
7. How should the desired types of personnel be educated?

Recommendations for geriatric training to date have been more qualitative than quantitative. This book explores both quality and qantity and
examines implications of the several strategies proposed for meeting the
health-care needs of the elderly. Our focus is on physician services.

We use the term *geriatrics* in this book to describe the work of a geriatrician or his surrogate. As will be developed in chapter 3, we view the geriatrician as the physician who provides most of the care for illness of all kinds
in the elderly. A major component of care for the elderly is in the area of
mental illness. The geriatric psychiatrist is alternatively referred to as a
geropsychiatrist or a *psychogeriatrician*.

Customarily, the term *elderly* is linked to an arbitrarily assigned age,
usually 65. In a changing society, this cutoff point has become anachronis-
tic (Federal Council on Aging 1978). We recognize that labeling a class of
people on the basis of a single characteristic such as age is misleading.
Undoubtedly the elderly are heterogeneous in terms of their functional
capacity and their demands for health care. Nonetheless, most available
data have been collected by age group. Since the time of Bismarck, and
especially since the advent of Social Security, "65 years and older" has
become an important age category. Because the age cutoff of 65 does not
correspond to frailty, when possible we have used smaller increments of age
to distinguish the "young-old" (65 to 74 years) from the "old-old" (over 75
years).

An Ideal Model

An analysis of manpower needs depends on three elements: (1) a specifica-
tion of the goals to be achieved, (2) the current level of achievement *such*

that (1) minus (2) estimates the size of the task, and (3) the efficiency of different groups of manpower in meeting the task. In the case of geriatric manpower estimation, we are bereft of critical information and therefore need to compromise our strategy for projecting needs.

Reasonably strong consensus can be reached about goals for the health care of the elderly. Although terminology may vary with disciplinary or philosophic background, most observers agree with the following goals:

1. *Maximizing the independence of the individual.* This includes the ability to function physically and mentally at a level that would permit as much self-care as possible and some minimal threshold of economic and social support.
2. *Ensuring at least a minimal level of comfort.* This concept goes beyond the absence of severe pain to include attempts to lessen the anxiety and depression associated with functional limitations, disease states, and losses of role and relationship.
3. *Promoting subjective well-being or morale.* Despite the high prevalence of chronic illness, symptoms can be alleviated and the sense of physical and mental "wellness" heightened. Subjective well-being and morale are ambitious goals of a health-care system and are perhaps inappropriate if taken out of context. Yet, because health care of the elderly is often an indeterminate (as opposed to time-limited) activity, and because its ministrations are often intrusive on the life-style of the patient, a secondary goal of health-care providers is the issue of subjective well-being.
4. *Avoiding premature death.* Although mortality is inevitable, correctable problems contributing to mortality should be recognized and treated. Even if we cannot achieve the 100 years imputed as the "natural" human lifespan, we should be able to avoid those causes of death that are amenable to treatment.
5. *Minimizing the cost of care for the elderly.* Some political scientists have commented on the potentially disruptive societal effects of an inordinate public investment in the elderly to the detriment of other needy sectors (Hudson 1978). Others argue that the United States still spends proportionately less than other Western nations (Wilensky 1975). In either case, the objective is to achieve the first four goals at the least cost possible by avoiding waste and searching for efficient solutions.

Achievement of the first four goals requires the use of health personnel to treat patients in four categories.

1. *Acutely ill.* The acutely ill patient requires the diagnosis and treatment

of disease, the provision of comforting and caring services, and the mobilization of related ancillary services.

2. *Chronically ill, noninstitutionalized.* These patients need the same general classes of services as the acutely ill, but with much more emphasis on the mobilization of all health-care and social-support resources.

3. *Chronically ill, institutionalized.* Chronically ill patients require the same classes of services as the first two categories; but there is an additional need to assess the effect on care of the institutional environment, which is a part of the price of that care.

4. *"Well."* This group may require preventive care, both primary and secondary, including detection of asymptomatic disease, and may also need services to promote or maintain social functioning.

Our data are insufficient for us to itemize the individual services that pertain to each of these groups. Nor can we describe conclusively how the provision of an aliquot of service would increase the status of a given individual toward one or more of the goals outlined. Our limited knowledge base does suggest, however, that the relationship between services and outcomes is not linear. Marginal calculations must be used to estimate increments of benefits and costs.

Because of present knowledge gaps, even drawing on expert judgments, we cannot pursue the manpower-planning strategy proposed by the Graduate Medical Education National Advisory Committee (GMENAC 1979). This approach requires empirical data to estimate satisfactorily both the service needs and their manpower implications. We must fall back on simpler, but admittedly cruder, data on utilization patterns rather than effectiveness. In acknowledging this step, we identify the first of several important areas for needed future research.

Extrapolating from utilization patterns allows us to add a quantitative dimension to the manpower requirements implied by the qualitative recommendations of the IOM. These projections, in turn, provide a basis for formulating a series of alternative strategies for meeting manpower needs.

To develop estimates of physician manpower needed for the care of the elderly, we examined the actual and potential contributions of geriatric medical specialists; primary-care physicians (general practice, family practice, and general internal medicine); medical subspecialists; psychiatrists; and geropsychiatrists. We did not attempt estimates of the need for general-surgical and surgical-specialty, gynecologic, radiologic, pathologic, rehabilitative, ophthalmologic, or other similar manpower. These large groups are omitted, not because they in any way eschew participation in the care of the elderly, but rather because neither society nor the medical profession perceives a need for subgroups in these fields with special competence in geriatrics. Thus we postulate, essentially without dissent, that the foreseeable future will not witness the emergence of geriatric surgeons, geriatric gynecologists, or the like. On the other hand, medical specialists and primary-care providers for the elderly may indeed need additional knowledge and skill in geriatrics in order to relate appropriately to those surgical specialists most involved in treating the elderly (such as ophthalmologists, orthopedists, and urologists).

As the fraction of the aged in the population rises, representation of the elderly in the practice of these various specialists will also grow. The only implication of this prediction for manpower policy is that the need for those specialists who treat a disproportionate number of elderly patients will assuredly increase. For example, the aging of the population will increase the need for expert care of cataracts and hence for ophthalmologists, and for care of fractures and hence for orthopedists. Policymakers should take note of these possibilities when they consider curtailment of training in certain surgical subspecialties. This, however, is not within our self-assigned research area. Rather, this book focuses on ways of meeting the needs of the elderly for primary care and for the type of specialized backup that might be provided by internal medicine and its subspecialties and by psychiatry. It is here that the most challenging policy issues are concentrated.

This report may be challenged as being too readily cast in the familiar medical model consistent with physician preeminence. We hasten to emphasize that we do not imply a preference for the medical model of care for the elderly over one that is more socially oriented. In fact, we suggest that the present distinction between these two approaches is counterproductive. Comprehensive care for the elderly requires a synthesis of both.

It is indeed possible to consider a very different system of care in which social, rather than medical, professionals are the dominant actors and physicians are called in as technical experts on physiologic matters. However, such a shift may present a host of different problems. As we will endeavor to describe, geriatrics is a neglected area in this country. A proposal to transfer responsibility away from the physician may be misconstrued as an opportunity for the physician to abrogate responsibility in an area where more, not fewer, skills are needed. Moreover, the presence of physician leadership (but not necessarily physician dominance) can do much to augment the power and prestige of caring for the elderly. This consideration will become increasingly important as the competition for human-services funds grows keener.

Although we focus on issues surrounding physician manpower and possible substitutes for it, we imply no disregard for the variety of health professionals who can and do care for the elderly in very important ways. In other studies, our methods might be profitably applied to analysis of the need for other geriatric personnel. We note, however, that the data currently available on many of these professions are far less complete than those for physicians.

In summary, our subject is an analysis of the implications of different manpower configurations for meeting projected future needs for geriatric medical services. We examine the needs for geriatric manpower by combining an analysis of available data on geriatric-physician needs with an assessment of some of the strategies that might be considered in responding to the demographic imperative. We recognize that the training of needed geriatric personnel will require the development of new tools and that the effective deployment of these personnel will necessitate changes in certain rules and regulations that currently preclude or restrain such activities. These steps are also addressed in this book.

The Remainder of the Book

In chapter 2, the anticipated changes in the geriatric population and its utilization of health-care resources are examined. Against this backdrop, we present data about the current supply of geriatric manpower and the behavior of physicians currently treating the elderly. We also discuss the current signs of medical educators' interest in developing an increased emphasis on the elderly in the training of physicians.

Chapter 3 describes the debate on how best to increase physician attention to the care of the elderly. The roles of geriatric specialists and primary-care physicians are compared, and the potential substitutive contributions that might be made by nonphysician health practitioners are discussed. Also in chapter 3, we develop a series of physician manpower configurations. In a later chapter, we present quantitative projections of manpower for each scenario.

The next several chapters deal with geriatric-manpower projections. In chapter 4 we estimate the need for academic geriatricians. Chapter 5 outlines the several methods used for estimating the need for geriatric manpower and presents the results of our quantitative geriatric-manpower analysis when the several configurations of care are translated into numbers. Because the rather detailed discussion of the technical methods employed may not be interesting to the casual reader but is important for an appreciation of the kinds of assumptions that had to be made in developing boundary estimates, it is provided as appendix B. Chapter 6 describes our estimates of the need for geropsychiatrists in both academic and practice roles.

Chapter 7 examines the implications of our calculations with particular attention to issues not included in the model. Here we describe various ways in which health-care personnel might be deployed and the kind of health-care settings that might be developed to provide the best care to the elderly. The problems of recruiting practitioners into the field of geriatrics are discussed in terms of barriers and disincentives that militate against an effective manpower policy. The issue of whether geriatrics should be a specialty is approached through analogies drawn from the historical evolution of pediatrics and family practice as specialty areas.

Chapter 8 addresses the launching of a geriatric training program. Strategies for the introduction of new curricular content are described, and a model set of education objectives is offered. We conclude with some specific problems that are anticipated and with proposed solutions.

Chapter 9 concerns the challenge of measurement, discussing the selection of tools that might be used by practicing geriatricians to support patient care and research. Special attention is given to the criteria for choosing instruments, with emphasis on the purpose of the measurement. The importance of general measurements of functional status emerges from our need to evaluate our effectiveness in achieving the several goals of geriatrics listed previously on either an individual or a group basis. Chapter 9 develops the rationale for measurement in geriatrics, whereas a forthcoming volume (Kane and Kane 1981) discusses available instruments by content categories and makes recommendations for instrument choices.

Chapter 10 describes research goals for the development of a new and necessary fund of knowledge to improve the care of the elderly. The emphasis here is on topics in the area of clinical and health services research rather than of biomedical research. Although beyond the scope of our project, the latter subject was thoroughly treated in the IOM report and other recent writings. Our inclusion of health services research lies in its importance for the development of national policy in the coming decades.

The final chapter offers a set of recommendations related to the spectrum of geriatric needs outlined in this book.

2 Present Status of Health Care of the Elderly

Inexorable demographic trends have produced a rapid increase in the geriatric age group in this country, and projections are for still greater increases as the current cohorts age. This growth has a discernible impact on the utilization of health care. Against this background, the number of currently available physicians with geriatric competence is inadequate. More encouraging is the evidence that medical-educational institutions are beginning to respond to the demographic shifts by developing new curricula.

The Demographic Imperative

An overview of demographic and economic trends is a prerequisite for forecasting future needs or demands for medical care of the elderly. More detailed data are available from our source materials, particularly Kovar's studies (Kovar 1977a, 1977b).

The number of aged persons in the United States has been growing rapidly, both in absolute terms and relative to the total population. The numbers of the aged and their percentage of the total population are shown in table 2-1 for selected years. Projections for 1990 and beyond must assume changes in death rates and (for estimations of the total population) changes in birth rates. The projections shown in table 2-1 are based on an assumed gradual decrease in death rates from their 1976 levels; the figures would change significantly if death rates from heart disease, cancer, or stroke were to decrease dramatically.

Decreasing death rates have had some effect on the elderly population explosion, but past birth rates are more important. Table 2-2 shows the birth rate per 1,000 at selected critical points. The fluctuations in the birth rate are seen 65 years later in the numbers of "young-old" (aged 65 to 74) and 75 years later in the numbers of "old-old." Thus, following the birth rate, the numbers of elderly will grow rapidly until about 1990, level off as the Depression babies age, and then grow explosively after 2010 when the postwar baby boom arrives. Only then will the percentage of aged overtake

---

Detailed and current information on population projections through 2050 can be found in *Current Population Reports,* Series P-25. Other characteristics of the current population are reported in Series P-20 and P-60. Population and economic trends are surveyed and interpreted in Clark, Kreps, and Spengler (1978).

Table 2-1
The Aged in the United States: Trends

Age Group	Year						
	1910	1940	1970	1977	1990[a]	2010[a]	2030[a]
Population (millions)							
65+	4.0	9.0	20.0	23.4	29.8	34.8	55.0
65-74	2.8	6.4	12.4	14.6	17.8	19.7	31.8
75+	1.2	2.6	7.6	8.8	12.0	15.1	23.2
Percentage of total population							
65+	4.3	6.8	9.9	10.8	12.3	12.6	18.3
65-74	3.0	4.8	6.1	6.7	7.3	7.1	10.6
75+	1.3	2.0	3.8	4.1	5.0	5.5	7.7

Source: U.S. Department of Commerce, Bureau of the Census, *1970 Census of the Population*, 1973.

[a] Assuming (1) a fertility level of 2.1 children born per woman and (2) a decrease in mortality rates at a rate whereby life expectancy at birth increases by about 0.05 year per year.

Table 2-2
Birth Rate Per 1,000 U.S. Population

Year	Birth Rate
1905	31
1920	28
1935	19
1950	25
1965	20
1977	15

Sources: U.S. DHEW, *Vital Statistics of the U.S., Vol. 1* (1970); U.S. DHEW, *Health, United States, 1978,* Publication no. (PHS) 78–1282 (1978).

the levels above 13 percent that stable European countries such as Britain, France, and Sweden have today.

Recently, women have made greater gains in longevity than men. This is shown in table 2–3, which gives life expectancies by sex and race for selected years. Note that since 1900, 60-year-old white men have gained only 2.5 years in life expectancy, whereas women have gained 6.8 years. Demographers expect these longevity differences to persist. The result, seen in table 2–4, is that the proportion of women in older age groups has

Table 2-3
Life Expectancy at Ages 20 and 60, by Sex and Race

| | Life Expectancy, Age 20 | | | | Life Expectancy, Age 60 | | | |
| | Male | | Female | | Male | | Female | |
Year	White	Other	White	Other	White	Other	White	Other
1900	42	35	44	37	14.4	12.6	15.2	13.6
1940	48	40	51	42	15.1	14.4	17.0	16.1
1970	50	44	57	52	16.1	15.4	20.8	19.0
1976	52	47	59	55	16.9	16.3	22.0	20.7

Sources: U.S. DHEW, *Vital Statistics of the United States, Vol 2* (1973); U.S. DHEW, *Monthly Vital Statistics, Final Mortality Statistics, 1976* (1978).

Table 2-4
Proportion of the Aged That Are Female

| | Percentage | | |
Age Group	1940	1977	1990
65-74	50	56	56
75+	53	64	65

Source: U.S. Department of Commerce, Bureau of the Census, *Current Population Reports,* Series P-25 (1977).

increased. Moreover, the sex ratio for older people inevitably affects marital status, as shown in table 2-5. The sex ratio should be stable for the foreseeable future.

Living arrangements of the aged have been changing rapidly, partly because of the somewhat improved economic status of the elderly, and perhaps also because of changes in tastes of the elderly and their relatives. A recent survey has shown that over 50 percent of adults think it a "bad idea" for older parents to live with children (U.S. Department of Commerce 1977d). As table 2-6 shows, the proportion of aged persons in institutions (mainly nursing homes) has increased dramatically since 1960. The proportion of old people living with their families (other than their spouses) has declined. In 1940, 16 percent of aged men and 29 percent of aged women were living in households with a relative (usually a child) as head; this was reduced in 1975 to 4 and 12 percent, respectively. The combined effect of the sex differential in longevity and the change in living groupings is that 37 percent of elderly women are now living alone. This trend will be reinforced

Table 2-5
Proportion of the Aged That Are Married

	Percentage Married			
	1940		1977	
Age Group	Male	Female	Male	Female
65–74	69	42	80	50
75+	50	18	69	22

Source: U.S. Department of Commerce, Bureau of the Census, *Current Population Reports,* Series P-20 (1977).
Note: Inmates of institutions are excluded from these figures.

Table 2-6
Residential Status of the Aged

	Percentage in Residential Status			
	1960		1975	
Residential Status	Male	Female	Male	Female
Married, spouse present	67	35	73	36
Other head of family	6	12	3	8
In family, not head	9	21	4	12
Primary individual	13	27	15	37
Secondary individual	3	3	1	1
In institution	2	2	4	6

Source: U.S. Department of Commerce, Bureau of the Census, *Social Indicators, 1976;* U.S. Department of Commerce, Bureau of the Census, *Current Population Reports,* Series P-20 (1977).

by the drop in fertility that occurred during the 1930s. The next cohort of women is more likely to be childless or to have fewer children with whom to live. Because blacks tend to have larger families and to be poorer, they are more likely to be living with relatives. Despite the financial incentive for old couples to live together without getting married, the percentage of households with two unrelated persons of opposite sex has declined in recent years among the aged.

The aged poor are being left behind in declining central cities and impoverished rural districts, where they are often ill served. Continued migration to the major sun-belt centers in Florida, Southern California, and the Southwest keeps the aged population high in these areas.

The elderly remain poorer than the middle aged; their relative position has remained constant despite the fact that their real income has doubled since World War II. Such in-kind subsidies as Medicare, Medicaid, food stamps, subsidized housing, and Social Security entitlements for survivors make it difficult to measure the effective income of the aged poor. For example, public contributions to health expenditures per elderly person were over $1,000 in 1976. These services are presumably not worth $1,000 to the recipient (that is, if given the money instead of the services, recipients might decide to spend some of it on something else) but may well be worth a large fraction of that amount. Indicators of improving economic position include earlier retirement and greater ability to live alone. In 1940, over half the men aged 65 to 74 were still working; but in 1976, this figure was only 20 percent. Currently, two-thirds of the workers covered by Social Security are choosing to retire before age 65 at the cost of reduced benefits.

Nonetheless, 15 percent of aged persons were below the official poverty level in 1975, although this was only about half the proportion found ten years earlier. Inflation has a disastrous effect on those with fixed savings or with pensions that are not tied to the cost of living. The median income of households with heads over age 65 in various categories in 1975 is compared with the same statistic for all households in table 2-7. Household income of the aged is about half the average overall, but household size is smaller and old people are more likely to own their homes outright. The personal income of aged men appears much higher than that of aged women ($5,500 versus $2,740 in 1975), but this is misleading because it does not treat Social Security retirement benefits as community property. In 1973 the surviving

Table 2–7
Median Income in 1975 of Households with Heads Over Age 65 and All Households

Type of Household	Households with Head over Age 65			All Households		
	Median Income (Dollars)	Mean Size	Percentage of Total	Median Income (Dollars)	Mean Size	Percentage of Total
All households	5,900	1.8	100	12,200	2.9	100
Owner occupied	6,700	1.9	71	14,600	3.1	64
Rented	4,400	1.5	29	8,700	2.4	36
One person	3,500	1.0	43	5,200	1.0	20
Husband–wife	8,500	2.3	46	15,300	3.5	65
Other	8,000	2.6	11	8,700	3.0	15

Source: U.S. Department of Commerce, Bureau of the Census, *Current Population Reports,* Series P-60 (1977).

spouse's share of Social Security benefits was raised to a full pension level. Thus, women in one-person households in 1974 had a median income of $2,900, which is 85 percent of the median income of men in the same situation.

Health Status and Utilization

A thorough review of the health status and associated use of medical-care services by the elderly is available elsewhere (Kover 1977b) and is beyond the scope of this project. Because these variables are important in assessing any estimate of manpower needs, however, a few points deserve special emphasis.

Health status is a difficult concept to assess. A person's expectations and environment affect his or her judgment about his own health. Thus it is possible to have almost 70 percent of the elderly noninstitutionalized population report their health as excellent (28 percent) or good (40 percent) while, at the same time, 85 percent suffer from at least one chronic condition and 47 percent are limited in activity because of chronic conditions (Kovar 1977b).

As shown by table 2-8, chronic illness and associated disability increase with age. Although all measures of activity restriction increase with age, the self-perception of wellness does not commensurately decrease as one passes from young-old to old-old. Most of the elderly view themselves as essentially well.

The elderly make consistently increased use of health services, with the exception of dental care (table 2-9). They see physicians about once more

Table 2-8
Chronic Illness and Associated Disability for Various Age Groups

Health Status	Age Group		
	45–64	65–74	75+
Number of chronic conditions per person	0.41[a]	0.65	0.87
Percentage limited in activity because of chronic conditions	24	42	56
Bed-disability days per year	9.3	10.3	17.4
Days of restricted activity per year	28.0	34.0	46.0
Percentage who perceived health as good or excellent	76[a]	69	68

Source: Composite data from the Health Interview Survey, U.S. DHEW National Center for Health Statistics, Series 10; and special analyses of NHIS data by Rand.
[a] Ages 55 to 59.

Table 2-9
Health-Service Utilization by Various Age Groups

	Age Group		
Health-Service Utilization	45–64	65–74	75+
Mean number of physician contacts per year	5.7	6.9	6.8
Mean number of dental visits per year	1.8	1.3	0.8
Percentage seeing a physician in past year	76[a]	80	81
Percentage seeing a dentist in past year	58.8	34.7	22.7
Nursing-home residents per 1000 persons	3.7	12	97.3[b]
Nonfederal hospital days per noninstitutionalized person	1.75	3.28	5.86
Operations per 1,000 persons	124.6	165.9[c]	

Sources: Composite data from the Health Interview Survey, U.S. DHEW National Center for Health Statistics, Series 10; and special analyses of NHIS data by Rand.

[a] Rate for ages 50 to 64.

[b] Rate for ages 75 to 84 = 58.9, and for 85+ = 236.6.

[c] Rate for ages 65+.

per year than those in the 45-to-64 age group, spend more than twice as much time in hospitals, and undergo one-third more surgical procedures. Of course, this greater utilization of services may not necessarily be due to greater demand instigated by consumer need; providers may indeed stimulate this pattern of consumption. The possible effects of insurance coverage (especially Medicare) are suggested by the low utilization of dental services, which are not covered under Medicare, and the leveling out of most other utilization after age 65 despite worsening health status. Not surprisingly, the most striking example of age-correlated utilization is in the use of nursing homes (nursing-home care is covered predominantly by Medicaid rather than Medicare). The proportion of people aged 75 and over in nursing homes is more than twenty-five times greater than in the 45-to-64 year age group.

Costs of Health-Care Spending

The high costs of health-care services have become a national concern, and the increase is most dramatic for the elderly. In 1977 the average health bill for those over 65 was $1,745, and 29 percent of the $142.6 billion spent by the country on health care was devoted to the aged (Gibson and Fisher 1979). Hospital-care expenditures for the aged rose from $3.7 billion in 1967 to $18.2 billion in 1977. Such trends have had a chilling effect on the expansion of new services and are pushing the debate on health care for the elderly from how many more resources are needed to how current resources might be used more effectively. (See, for example, Califano 1978; Hudson 1978; Binstock 1978; and Butler 1978.) Table 2-10 shows the per-capita expenditures for the elderly and the percentage publicly supported by type of service. Figure 2-1 compares total expenditures and source of funds for different age groups.[1]

Present Status of Geriatric Medicine

Despite the impressive amounts of money spent to purchase medical services for the elderly, there are few specialists in geriatric medicine in the United States and the field carries little prestige. We examine the current situation by analyzing available data on self-identified geriatricians in the United States and reviewing what information can be found that reflects the quality of the care rendered to the elderly today.

Self-Designated Geriatricians

The American Medical Association's 1977 survey of physicians' professional activities polled the 363,619 active practitioners with known

Table 2-10
Per-Capita Health-Care Expenditure for the Elderly and Source of Funds, by Type of Service
(*Year ending September 1977*)

Type of Service	Age 65 and Older		Ages 19-64	
	Total	Public	Total	Public
Per-capita expenditure	$1,745	$1,169	$661	$190
Hospital care	769	679	326	137
Nursing-home care	446	254	14	8
Physicians' services	302	180	159	22
Dentists' services	43	2	54	2
Other professional services	35	21	17	2
Drugs	121	18	58	4
Eyeglasses and appliances	13	a	12	1
Other health services	16	15	21	13

Source: R.M. Gibson and C.R. Fisher, "Age Differences in Health Care Spending, Fiscal Year 1977," *Social Security Bulletin* 42(1979): table 1 (entries are rounded to the nearest dollar).
a Less than $0.50.

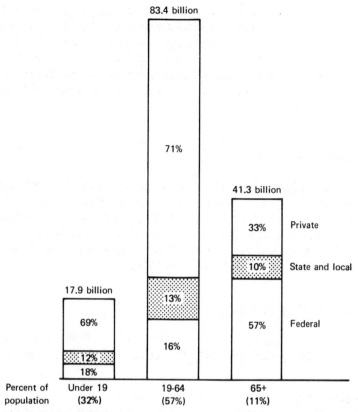

Source: R.M. Gibson and C.R. Fisher, "Age Differences in Health Care Spending, Fiscal Year 1977," *Social Security Bulletin* 42(1979):3–16.

Figure 2–1. Percentage Distribution of Health-Care Expenditures, by Source of Funds, for Three Age Groups, Fiscal-Year 1977

addresses, receiving an 88-percent response rate. As part of the study, the physicians were asked to designate the number of hours they spent per week in the activities related to one or more specialties. Consequently, in the AMA physician master file, physicians may be classified by as many as three self-identified specialties that are further broken down into primary, secondary, and tertiary specialties in order of perceived time commitment. The AMA has made available to us a tape containing descriptive data on all physicians who indicated geriatrics as a primary, secondary, or tertiary specialty in the 1977 survey. Comparison data on the total population of physicians were drawn from *Physician Distribution and Medical Licensure in the United States, 1977* (Goodman 1979). When a particular item was not available from this source, we used the most recent year for which the desired datum could be found in *Profile of Medical Practice, 1978* (Gaffney 1979).

The prevalence of geriatrics as a self-reported specialization is shown in table 2–11; this field was listed as the primary specialty by 371, as secondary by 187, and as tertiary by 71, for a total of 629 individuals. Assuming an 88-percent response rate, this would be equivalent to 715 physicians out of 363,619, or 0.2 percent. Those who listed geriatrics as the primary specialty most commonly considered their secondary specialty to be general or family practice, internal medicine, psychiatry, general surgery, or orthopedic surgery; 125 indicated geriatrics as a sole specialty interest. Among those whose secondary specialty was geriatrics, the primary specialty was most often internal medicine, general or family practice, psychiatry, or emergency medicine. Taken together, the 629 who cited geriatrics at all, additionally listed common specialties of general or family practice (201), internal medicine (144), and psychiatry (66). Curiously, 24 cited pediatrics! We can infer that slightly more than 10 percent of the self-identified geriatricians are also self-identified geropsychiatrists, 55 percent have branched into geriatrics from a primary-care field, and 20 percent consider themselves solely geriatricians (although they may have started as something else). The remaining 15 percent identify themselves with a wide variety of fields as well as with geriatrics.

Only one-quarter of the self-identified geriatricians were certified in any specialty as of December 1977, compared with a national average from the parent study of at least 49 percent, a minimal estimation based on figures for 1975. As an example, among 144 who listed themselves as internists, 40 were board certified. This is 28 percent, compared with a national average of 61 percent (a 1975 figure and therefore an underestimate). Seven geriatricians (1.1 percent) held board certification in two fields. Again, the national average for dual boards is higher (4 percent).

Data on society membership bore out much the same theme: 177 (28 percent) belonged to no professional societies. In order of frequency, membership in some societies of interest was as follows: American Geriatrics Society, 164 (26 percent); American College of Emergency Physicians, 130 (21 percent); American Academy of Family Physicians, 128 (20 percent); American College of Physicians, 32 (5 percent); American Psychiatric Association, 25 (4 percent); and American College of Surgeons, 18 (3 percent). Clearly, the geriatricians were neither academicians nor joiners. Only 3 belonged to societies for clinical research. The average geriatrician belonged to only 1.2 professional societies. Qualitatively, the surprising finding was the large number of geriatricians who were members of the American College of Emergency Physicians (ACEP). Only 20 had indicated emergency medicine as a first, second, or third specialty, yet 130 belonged to the College. The connection between geriatrics and the ACEP is unclear, unless a significant number of individuals are dividing their time between tours of emergency duty and a geriatric practice. Among those whose primary specialty was geriatrics, an even higher percentage (28) belonged to the

Table 2–11
Physicians' Self-Perceived Specialization in Geriatrics

	Number of Physicians
Geriatrics is physicians' primary specialty	371
Physicians' secondary specialty: [a]	
General practice or family practice	80
Internal medicine	51
Psychiatry	19
General surgery	13
Orthopedic surgery	12
No secondary specialty	125
Geriatrics is physicians' secondary specialty	187
Physicians' primary specialty: [b]	
General practice or family practice	63
Internal medicine	41
Psychiatry	22
Emergency medicine	12
Geriatrics is physicians' tertiary specialty	71
Total physicians interested in geriatrics	629 (or 0.2% of respondents)

Source: American Medical Association Physician Masterfile, December 1977.

[a] Total of subcolumn does not add to 371 because less frequently mentioned (10 or less) secondary specialties combined with geriatrics are excluded.

[b] Total does not add to 187 because less frequently mentioned (10 or less) primary specialties combined with geriatrics are excluded.

ACEP, suggesting that emergency medicine was most likely to be a secondary interest.

As might be anticipated, the geriatricians were older than the average American physician (table 2–12). The median age was 56 for active geriatricians and 49 for all physicians, whether active or not. The median year of graduation from medical school for geriatricians was 1948; the median year of licensure to practice was 1955. The data in table 2–12 dramatize the relative absence from the geriatric ranks of residents and recent graduates from residency. They also show the tendency to enter geriatrics as a result of "aging with one's patients." About 20 percent of geriatricians were 65 to 74 years of age (versus 9.2 percent among all physicians). Moreover, the 4.9 percent of geriatricians aged 75 and older includes active physicians only, whereas the 4.3-percent figure for all physicians over 75 includes those who are inactive, are unclassified, or have unknown addresses. The latter group is likely to include a disproportionate number of elderly, making the relative proportion of geriatricians over age 75 even more discrepant with practice trends. The sex distribution of geriatricians closely parallels that for the general physician population.

Table 2-12
Age Distribution of Geriatricians Compared with All Physicians, December December 31, 1977

Age	Geriatricians, Frequency (%)	All Physicians, Frequency (%)
Under 35	5.6	27.3
35–44	19.0	24.7
45–54	22.5	20.1
55–64	28.7	14.4
65–74	19.3	9.2
75 +	4.9	4.3
Total	100.0	100.0
N	629	421,278[a]

[a]This frequency distribution is based on all physicians, including those who were inactive or not classified and whose addresses were unknown.

The AMA survey affords only a glimpse into the practice profile of the geriatrician. Office-based patient care was indicated by 65 percent as their major professional activity, and 25 percent chose hospital-based patient care. Teaching (0.8 percent) and research (1.1 percent) were rare, confirming the inference from the society-membership data. None of the 629 were inactive or retired; although 43 were in administration, only 4 were in other non-patient-care activities.

These data from the AMA master file confirm what others have suggested: Most of the care of the elderly falls to those who do not perceive themselves as geriatricians, especially the primary-care providers such as the general internist and the family practitioner. Furthermore, the few who do view themselves as geriatricians have minimal formal credentials.

Measures of Physician Practice

Two sources of data can be drawn on for insight into aspects of physician practice. The first is the National Ambulatory Medical Care Survey (NAMCS), a recurrent data set compiled by the National Center for Health Statistics from encounter forms completed by a randomly selected cross-section of physicians (Tenney, White, and Williamson 1974). As the name implies, it is limited to ambulatory care only (essentially office and outpatient-based care). The second source of data on physician activities was collected by the University of Southern California School of Medicine's Division of Research in Medical Education (USC/DRME 1978) as part of a one-time nationwide study of practicing physicians in more than twenty medical and surgical specialties. Using the AMA data base, the USC/DRME team drew a stratified random sample of each specialty. Log diaries were maintained by each participating physician for each of two three-day periods. All activities were covered, and specific data were recorded about patients seen. The central objectives of the USC/DRME studies were to obtain national measures within and between selected specialty groups on (1) how physicians spend their professional and nonprofessional time; (2) the types of patients seen and the characteristics of both the encounter and the service rendered; and (3) the relationships of practice, organizational factors, geographic location, and community characteristics with physician activities (Mendenhall, Girard, and Abrahamson 1978; Mendenhall et al. 1978).

Because the USC/DRME studies cover a broader spectrum of physician activities than does the NAMCS, we have chosen to use the former as a major data source for the present project and to use NAMCS data, when available, for independent verification. In some instances, we have contracted with USC/DRME for special analyses of their data to address aspects of geriatric care not otherwise covered in their reports.[2]

For purposes of estimating utilization, we have not considered the surgical specialties because we do not anticipate that the geriatrician would have a direct or potential replacement role in those areas. We have also chosen to treat psychiatric care separately in another part of this report (chapter 6).

Data from the USC/DRME studies on encounters with elderly patients on a typical day for physicians in primary care and medical specialties are given in table 2-13. As shown, primary-care providers account for most of the care. Family and general practitioners provide the largest segment of nonhospital care, and general internists the largest fraction of hospital visits. Among medical specialists, cardiologists see most of the elderly patients; dermatologists see the next-largest number of outpatients; and neurologists, chest physicians, and gastroenterologists treat the next-largest number of inpatients.

Conversely, data from the USC/DRME studies show that, as a percentage of total encounters, patients 65 years and older account for 35 percent of visits to internists, 35 percent of visits to family physicians (including general practitioners), and 6 percent of visits to psychiatrists. These proportions are closely approximated in data from the NAMCS for outpatient visits only.

Physician Aversion to Care of the Elderly

If medical manpower especially trained for and interested in the care of the elderly is scarce, the next question is: How attentive and considerate are

Table 2-13
National Estimates of Physician–Patient Encounters per Day, by Physician Specialty, Setting, and Patient Age

Physician Specialty	Nonhospital Encounters per Day				Hospital Encounters per Day			
	Number Aged 65–74	Percentage	Number Aged 75+	Percentage	Number Aged 65–74	Percentage	Number Aged 75+	Percentage
Internal medicine	56,114	32	36,522	30	46,740	48	46,076	48
General practice	75,692	43	57,048	47	22,723	23	26,869	28
Family practice	17,547	10	13,492	11	6,096	6	7,450	8
Cardiology	9,823	6	5,271	4	9,442	10	7,393	8
Dermatology	7,786	4	4,192	3	451	—	320	—
Pulmonology	1,886	1	1,043	1	2,839	3	1,520	2
Gastroenterology	1,711	1	921	1	2,415	2	1,714	2
Hematology	943	—	508	—	1,316	1	933	1
Oncology	624	—	227	—	796	1	365	1
Allergy	1,484	1	799	1	223	—	159	—
Rheumatology	971	—	523	—	498	—	354	—
Neurology	1,336	1	720	1	3,035	3	2,153	2
Endocrinology	442	—	238	—	497	—	352	—
Infectious disease	146	—	78	—	306	—	217	—
Nephrology	635	—	342	—	753	1	534	—

Source: Practice Study Reports (USC/DRME data), table 2.2.1, Board Certified and Nonboard Certified.
Note: Unpublished data were available for the two age intervals in internal medicine, general practice, family practice, cardiology, pulmonology, and oncology. The remaining categories were estimated by applying the average proportions of those aged 75+ (35 percent nonhospital, 50 percent hospital) of the three medical specialties: cardiology, pulmonology, and oncology for the figures available for age 65+. There was no basis from which to estimate the age distribution of encounters for obstetrics-gynecology or otohinolaryngology.

generalist, nonspecialized, nongeriatric physicians? This is obviously a difficult question to answer. Anecdotes from patients and the parlance of young physicians ("crock," "turkey," "gomer") certainly suggest that attentiveness to the elderly is less than that accorded to younger persons; but such data may fail to reflect the experiences and attitudes of a putative "silent majority."

Although a substantial part of the workload of primary-care providers is devoted to the care of the elderly, some evidence suggests that these tasks are not pursued avidly. Studies of physician visits to nursing-home patients show a consistent pattern of minimal care (Solon and Greenawalt 1974; U.S. Senate 1975). Care given tends to be brief and often superficial, with a conspicuous absence of complete examinations or active attention to therapy (Kane, Hammer, and Byrnes 1977). Physician attention appears to be due more to a response to federal regulations than to a commitment to the nursing-home patients (Willemain 1979). A particularly poignant statement by a patient, which identifies all too clearly the effects of such physician behavior, appeared in the *Los Angeles Times* in September 1979 and is reproduced as appendix A.

Because the nursing-home resident may not be viewed as a highly desirable patient, one might have expected that office and hospital practice would reflect a different style. The elderly patient is often afflicted with a variety of chronic diseases and presents the physician with multiple problems. It would have seemed reasonable to hypothesize that office and hospital contacts with them would, if anything, be longer than those with younger patients. Therefore, we turned to the data of the USC/DRME study of the practice patterns of various types of physicians and examined the encounter time (face to face between doctor and patient) as a function of the patient's age. Our hypothesis was that physicians of all types would spend more time with elderly patients than with middle-aged adults for all types of encounters because the elderly are alleged to take longer to prepare for examination and to comprehend the physician's explanation of diagnosis and treatment. To our surprise, average encounter time declined as a function of age.

The results of our calculations are based on the comparison of weighted mean encounter times for patients of different ages. These weighted means were not computed from the raw data on encounter times gathered in the USC study, but from tabulated mean encounter times for each specialty, age group, location, and visit-characteristics category. A list of the range of each dimension appears in table 2-14. In all, we used $7 \times 4 \times 2 \times 15 = 840$ means.

To find whether our final differences are significant, we need to know the error of estimate of each of the 840 means. This was derived from a model of the distribution of encounter time in the original data. For a fixed

Table 2-14
Dimensions of the Array of Encounter-Time Means

Specialty	Patient Age Group	Location	Classification
Cardiology	45–54	Hospital	All
Family practice	55–64	Nonhospital	Type:
Gastroenterology	65–74		First
General practice	75 +		Episodic
			Principal care
Internal medicine			Consultative
Oncology			Specialized
			Severity:
			None
			Minor
Pulmonology			Moderate
			Severe
			Complexity:
			Minimal
			Brief
			Limited
			Extended
			Comprehensive

specialty and location category, let t_{ai} be the encounter time of person i in age group a. We assume that

$$t_{ai} = E(t) + d_a + e_{ai},$$

where

$E(t)$ = the average value of t_{ai} over all ages and individuals.

d_a = the shift due to age.

e_{ai} = an independent, identically distributed variable with mean 0 and standard deviation s.

We can estimate s from a breakdown of visits in each category by length of visit. It was always between 15 and 20 minutes in a sample of medical categories. In principle, this standard deviation can be reduced somewhat by controlling for encounter type, severity, or complexity. In fact, encounter times did not differ much for different type or severity of episodes, so that the within-characteristic variance remained large. Encounter times did vary substantially by complexity, so that the standard deviation within complexity types was somewhat smaller, between 13 and 15 minutes in a sample.

The standard error of estimate of any of the 840 means is the standard deviation of the individual encounter times divided by the number of encounters in the sample. The estimated number of encounters with patients

Table 2-15
Sample Encounters by Specialty and Location

Specialty	Mendenhall Study Population	Number Interviewed	Estimated Encounters with Patients 45 + [a]	
			Nonhospital	Hospital
Cardiology	6,453	297	4,500	4,500
Family practice	9,000[b]	504	11,500	3,500
Gastroenterology	2,033	249	2,600	3,100
General practice	40,600[b]	328	7,500	2,000
Internal medicine	37,000[b]	739	12,500	10,000
Oncology	400[b]	218	3,000	3,500
Pulmonology	1,951	208	2,200	3,000

[a] Estimated by reducing national population estimates by fraction of specialty interviewed.
[b] Estimated by subdividing tabulated category.

45 and older for each specialty-location category is shown in table 2-15. It is derived by dividing the national weights provided by the USC/DRME study by the national specialty population sampled, and then multiplying by the number of that specialty actually interviewed and the number of days (3) they kept a diary.

Since the big difference in encounter times is between patients under 65 and patients over 65, most of our comparisons are between those age groups. Given a total sample of N, the standard error of the difference is smallest when the groups are equal in size, when it equals $s/(1/N/2 + 1/N/2)^{1/2}$.

Since the seven specialties under study provide most of the medical care of the elderly, we can combine their experience to get an idea of the overall experience. The specialties were weighted by the fraction of overall encounters provided to patients 45 and over. The error in the combination is given by

$$s(\sum N_i^2/n_i)^{1/2}/N$$

where

i indexes the specialties.

n_i represents the encounters in the sample.

N_i represents the average daily encounters for patients over 45 in the ith speciality.

$N = \sum N_i$.

This error is dominated by the categories that were lightly sampled in the USC/DRME study, namely general practice and internal medicine (for nonhospital encounters) and internal medicine (for hospital encounters).

Differences in encounter times between age groups might be due to differences in the mix of complexity of cases. To control for this, we made comparisons on a standard case mix in addition to simple average comparisons. The case mix chosen for standardization was representative of most specialty–age group categories—for nonhospital: minimal 0.15, brief 0.3, limited 0.35, extended 0.15, comprehensive 0.05; for hospital, 0.2 in all five categories. Although the standard error within complexity types is generally about 20 percent less than the overall standard error of an age-specialty allocation category, the differences between the actual proportions in a category and the standard proportions increase the standard error of the standardized mean. The net effect is that comparisons controlling for complexity have only slightly smaller standard errors than uncontrolled comparisons. The main advantage of controlling for complexity is to correct for complexity differences between age groups.

The average encounter time for medical visits in and out of the hospital is shown in figure 2–2. In these results, the specialty averages are weighted by the fraction of overall encounters that that specialty produces, so that internal medicine, for example, counts much more heavily than oncology. As can be seen, the average encounter time rises slightly for 55- to 64-year-old patients, and then drops abruptly for 65- to 74-year-old patients, and slightly (insignificantly) more for the patients over 75. The big difference is between patients over and under 65. For this reason, and to simplify our presentation, in the rest of the chapter we report only differences between those under 65 and those 65 and over. The results are essentially the same whether the different age groups are adjusted to have the same complexity mix or not. The largest difference between the two methods is 0.3 minutes. The differences between younger and older patients are 1 minute for nonhospital encounters and 2 minutes for hospital encounters. These differences are highly significant.

The results differ from the "all"-encounters results of the USC/DRME survey because of standardization. For purposes of comparison, it seems better to standardize by complexity in order to remove the possible effects of case-mix differences and to isolate differences more directly attributable to age of patient; we will always do this.

There is a remarkable consistency across the seven medical specialties interviewed. Figure 2–3 shows the results. Each doctor type is represented by its initial on a graph. The horizontal coordinate gives the average encounter time for older patients, and the vertical coordinate gives the average encounter time for younger patients. If encounter times were equal, then the point would lie on the 45-degree line. As can be seen, for nonhos-

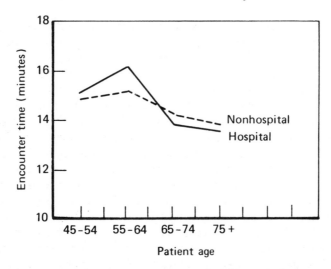

Note: Specialty times are weighted by their share of medical visits to obtain the overall average. Averages for different ages are standardized for complexity of cases.

Figure 2-2. Average Medical-Encounter Times by Age of Patient

pital visits all types are above the line, with cardiologists and pulmonologists showing the greatest differences and internists and general practitioners also significantly higher. For hospital encounters, general practitioners and the three subspecialist groups give approximately the same time to younger and older patients; but family practitioners, internists, and cardiologists give significantly more time to younger patients. Thus different medical specialties are consistent in giving less time per encounter to older patients both in and out of the hospital, but internists and cardiologists show the greatest overall differential.

When encounters are broken down by type, severity, and complexity, a new pattern emerges. Table 2-16 presents the results for the classes we considered. The second and fifth columns give the average difference in minutes for that type of visit, weighted by the number of visits that the physician specialty type sees. Although the times for all encounter classes except brief encounters and nonhospital first encounters are significantly shorter for older patients, the largest differences are in consultative and comprehensive visits. Presumably, these involve the most time-consuming and trickiest medical problems; either the visits of older patients are being classified differently, or dramatically less time is being taken for these difficult encounters.

Thus, any way the data are analyzed, it appears that physicians spend less time with elderly patients. The phenomenon might be due to frank pre-

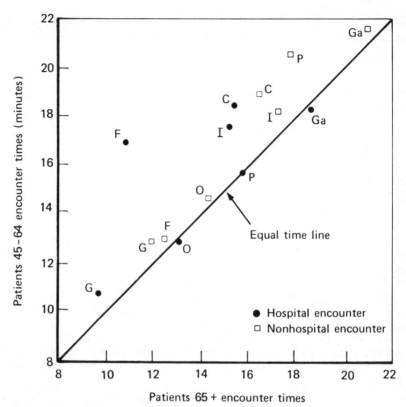

Note: C = cardiologists, F = family practitioners, G = general practitioners, Ga = gastro-enterologists, I = internists, O = oncologists, P = pulmonologists.

Figure 2–3. Encounter Time by Medical Specialty and Age of Patient

judice ("ageism"), but it might also be due to a reasoned, although quite possibly unjustified, analysis of relative priorities. For example, physicians may decide that they can accomplish more medical benefit by investing time in younger persons than in older ones in view of differences in reliability of history, compliance with directions, chronicity of complaints, responsiveness to therapy, and frequency of cures. In each of these characteristics, the elderly score lower than "average," although the degree of difference may be overblown in many physicians' minds (this in itself being another feature of ageism), aggravated by lack of awareness of ways to observe and measure progress of elderly patients.

In summary, although the underlying psychodynamics are matters for speculation, we offer some new data suggesting that there are more than

Table 2-16
Average Encounter Times by Encounter Type and Age of Patient

Encounter Classification	Nonhospital			Hospital		
	45–64	65+	z for Difference[a]	45–64	65+	z for Difference[a]
Severity						
Not severe	15.8	12.4	8	13.2	10.5	4
Moderately severe	15.5	14.3	6	14.3	12.4	8
Type						
First encounter	20.1	20.6	−1.5	20.8	18.1	4
Principal	13.9	13.1	5	13.2	12.5	3.5
Consultative	20.2	14.0	11	20.0	14.9	12
Extent						
Brief	10.8	11.1	−1.0	9.3	9.0	0.8
Extended	21.7	20.0	5	19.2	15.8	9
Comprehensive	33.9	26.7	12	26.3	22.7	9
Average scores						
Standardized average[b]	15.0	14.0	8	15.7	13.8	12
Raw average	14.9	13.7	9	15.8	13.7	13

[a] The standard errors for difference are assumed to be $sp^{1/2}$ minutes, where p is the proportion of total encounters represented by the type, and $s = 0.13$ for nonhospital, 0.16 for hospital. Values greater than 1.96 represent statistical significance at the .05 level; those greater than 2.57 at the .01 level.

[b] Standardized to a case mix of 15 percent minimal, 30 percent brief, 35 percent limited, 15 percent extended, and 5 percent comprehensive for nonhospital encounters, and to 20 percent each type for hospital encounters.

anecdotes to support the elderly's claims that they get short shrift from the medical profession.

Evidence of New Interest in Geriatrics

Medical Schools

A review of recently increasing efforts to solve at least one set of problems besetting the elderly—the shortage of health-care manpower with the interest and the ability to care for the special needs of the old—is encouraging. There are signs that a new vigor is replacing academic apathy. Focusing on the education of medical manpower, we find the first evidence of increased emphasis on aging in the 1970s. A review of medical-school catalogs for 1969 found the use of words referring to aging in 48 of 99 catalogs (Freeman 1971), but such phraseology was not translated into actual gerontologic curricular content. Meanwhile, Freeman reported only fifteen faculty positions in geriatrics or gerontology in medical schools across the entire country. The Senate Special Committee on Aging conducted brief questionnaire surveys of medical schools in 1971, 1974, and 1976. By 1976, of 87 schools responding, only 3 had established geriatrics "as a specialty in the curriculum" (Chicago Medical School, Arkansas College of Medicine, and University of North Dakota). The phrasing of the question, however, may have discouraged positive responses. Also in 1976, 43 percent of responding schools indicated that they offered opportunities for students, interns, or residents to serve in nursing homes; however, no information was provided on how frequently these options were elected or on the kinds of models of geriatric care supplied by the experience.

The 1976 survey of medical schools by Akpom and Mayer (1978) revealed a dearth of geriatric teaching. Although most of the medical schools reported offering geriatric material as an "elective in one form or another," the true geriatric content was scant and fragmentary and, for the most part, buried in other courses. Only 15 of the 96 respondent medical schools indicated that they taught geriatrics as a separate subject, and in only two was it a mandatory part of the curriculum. The August 1978 survey of medical schools by the Association of American Medical Colleges (AAMC) is quoted in the IOM report cited earlier. The survey showed a larger number of elective courses as a sign of increased activity, but attendance in these electives was low. Across the whole nation, only two mandatory free-standing courses on aging could be identified. There was some evidence of an increase in required rotations to nursing homes; 7 schools now reported this as mandatory, and 22 offered elective rotations to nursing homes. In contrast, by February 1979 (the same month the IOM report was released, although it was dated September 1978), Theodore Reiff was able to report in a newsletter that 46 medical schools "have or are developing geriatric medical programs."

In May 1979, the National Retired Teachers Association, the American Association of Retired Persons, and the George Washington University Medical Center cosponsored a conference in Washington, D.C. on geriatric medicine and medical-school/teaching-hospital responsibilities. In connection with this conference, the sponsors solicited material from all medical schools describing the status of their geriatric medical-education programs. Only 31 U.S. schools responded positively in writing, although many more than that sent representatives to the conference. Of the 31 schools, 17 reported mandatory curricular programs in gerontology and geriatrics. These ranged from four to twenty hours of lectures, seminars, and/or field trips during the first- or second-year courses. Only 2 schools reported mandatory geriatric clerkships. Many were planning new curricular offerings to begin in 1979–1980 or 1980–1981.

Most recently, the American Medical Student Association published its directory of clinical training sites for geriatrics, which also includes information on preclinical lecture courses (Coccaro 1979). By piecing together its information and combining it with the other findings, one can conclude that by June 1979 a total of 61 U.S. medical schools offered courses in geriatrics, gerontology, or both to medical students. Of these, 4 now mandate a clerkship in geriatric medicine or psychiatry and an additional 4 include geriatrics as part of a major clinical clerkship. In addition to these 8, another 21 intersperse didactic material in geriatrics or gerontology throughout the preclinical and clinical years as part of other courses. In 55 of the 61 schools, elective courses are offered; most of them are clinical clerkships of one kind or another.

Among the 63 U.S. medical schools not yet offering official courses on aging, stirrings of activity are occurring in at least 18. In these, at least one faculty member has been assigned responsibilities in geriatrics; and often an interdepartmental committee is analyzing the local situation with the aim of deciding how material on aging should be introduced into the curriculum. A reasonable projection would suggest that by mid-1980 there will be 80 schools with geriatric-gerontologic education programs. Once such a majority has been achieved, and recognizing the tendency of medical schools to conform to a "norm," we anticipate that all 124 schools will mount courses in gerontology and geriatrics for medical students, probably by 1995.

We conclude, therefore, that medical schools, for various reasons, are moving toward a consensus whereby most have recruited or will recruit geriatric faculty in departments of internal medicine, family practice, and/ or psychiatry. They have developed or will develop fifteen or more hours of gerontologic-geriatric teaching as a mandatory component of the first two years' curriculum. In most cases, these hours are presented as part of one or more courses that are more broadly oriented (Social Medicine, Behavioral Medicine, Community Medicine, Introduction to Clinical Medicine, Growth and Development). Clinical experience in geriatric medicine is less pervasive; generally it is either limited to field trips or elective, and the nursing home is the most common site for geriatric clerking. Even here, however, the trend seems to be toward increasing the clinical component and identifying a wider range of models of geriatric care for providing medical students with clinical exposure.

Why are medical schools now showing interest in geriatrics? The reasons are difficult to ascertain with certainty. In a few cases, legislative mandate and beneficence of state funding are key factors. Ohio is a prominent example. Others may be influenced by a desire to position themselves to be eligible for federal support should the Burdick bill or similar legislation be enacted. This bill would provide federal funds to support units (not necessarily departments) of geriatric medicine in medical schools. Its wellspring is a number of appeals from the academic community, exemplified in Pfeiffer's paper on the subject (1977). Federal agencies have also stimulated interest by supporting research (the National Institute on Aging) and fellowships in or affiliated with medical schools (the Veterans Administration (VA) and the Administration on Aging).

Immediate monetary stimuli do not appear to be the only cause of the change in the attitude of medical schools toward gerontology and geriatrics. The strongest additional reason is probably an appreciation of the changing demography of population and of health-care needs, as described earlier. Another reason is the growing emphasis on primary care in the curricula of many medical schools; geriatric medicine at the medical-student level can be viewed as the epitome of the science and practice of primary care. Nowhere in medicine can the importance of comprehensive concern for the patient as a person be more directly demonstrated than in geriatric medicine. Finally, there may be an element of pioneering in the medical schools' geriatric reorientation. With many decades of experience in hospital-based medical education and one decade of experience in ambulatory settings for teaching, the "last frontier" may be the development of teaching affiliations with such community geriatric facilities as multiservice centers, day hospitals, sheltered residences, and nursing homes.

Residencies and Fellowships

Geriatrics has surfaced in the academic medical centers not only in undergraduate medical-school curricula but also in residency and fellowship programs (Coccaro 1979). The IOM data-gathering group identified twenty-five residency programs in family practice that provide opportunities in geriatrics. These offerings are usually in the form of block-time rotations, but some provide opportunities for continuing care. Although figures are not available, we suspect that most of these rotations are elective rather than mandatory. Similarly, eighteen internal-medicine residencies have developed or will develop block-time rotations in geriatric medicine, and seven psychiatry residencies include from two to six months in geropsychiatry. The fellowship roster is changing rapidly. The twelve nationally authorized VA geriatric fellowship programs have all started within the past two years, each with two funded fellowship positions per class and a two-year program. Synthesizing data from the IOM report (1979) and the directory issued by the American Medical Student Association (Coccaro 1979), we found that as of June 1979, non-VA fellowship programs numbered seven in geriatric medicine and six in geropsychiatry, with two additional institutions having programs in both fields. In total, then, twenty-nine fellowship programs have been actuated for the 1979–1980 academic year. With an average capacity of two fellows per class, at full maturity, 58 fellows annually would finish programs and be available for academic or other positions. Our information is, however, that considerably fewer than 58 places have actually been filled in the 1979–1980 academic year. More recently, the Administration on Aging has funded a small number of fellowship programs to train faculty in geriatrics; but the graduates will provide fewer than fifteen new faculty members per year when the programs are fully operating.

Intensive developmental work is underway in health-care-educational circles. We have limited our description to schools of medicine as an example, lest this chapter become too long. There is a commensurate movement toward geriatrics and gerontology in nursing, dentistry, public health, and social welfare, as well as increasing attention to the problems of the elderly in schools of physical therapy, occupational therapy, podiatry, and speech and hearing specialties. It is this very ferment that stimulated the present study.

Notes

1. Further detail can be found in the annual articles by Gibson and Fisher on "Age Differences in Health Care Spending" in the *Social Security Bulletin* (for example, January 1979, pp. 3–16, and August 1977, pp. 3–14).

2. The Battelle Health and Population Study Center in Seattle has conducted a study of the reliability and validity of the data used in the USC/DRME project (Perrin, Harkins, and Marini 1978). Although that study identified a number of problems with regard to the data used to assess the primary-care components of practice, the more basic data used in this report were generally found to be reasonably reliable. One potential area of difficulty relates to estimates of physician contact time. Specific reliability studies on this variable were not possible, but numbers of visits and overall estimates of patient-contact time per day were reliable. One area, which may affect this measure, was shown to be very unreliable: time spent in nursing homes. Although physician time spent in nursing homes was about equally allocated by reporting physicians to either hospital or nonhospital services, the USC/DRME group had assumed that nursing-home time was assigned entirely to the nonhospital category. Thus, shorter contacts in the nursing home are somewhat overrepresented in hospital contact times. However, the volume of nursing-home care was sufficiently small to minimize the effect of this problem.

3 Rationale for Geriatric Manpower

In the preceding chapter, we described something of the plight of the elderly and adduced evidence hinting at poor quality of medical care. Now we turn to an examination of whether a change in medical manpower would be a promising strategy to improve the situation.

At least two lines of argument would militate against conscious development of new geriatric manpower. First, suggestions for new or additional manpower could be viewed as an encroachment on the territory of currently available categories of physicians. A different kind of argument is that geriatrics lacks an identifiable body of knowledge and thus requires no skills apart from those attained by any well-trained internist.

The Institute of Medicine (IOM) report has outlined the knowledge areas of geriatrics/gerontology. The geriatrician needs to be versed in the changes associated with aging and with the ranges of normal and abnormal responses attributable to those changes. To the degree that a variety of clinicians currently provide medical care to the elderly, they need to be aware of the ways in which the diagnostic and therapeutic procedures applicable to younger groups should be modified to conform to the epidemiologic and physiologic differences of an older population.

The geriatrician has specific knowledge of the variety of ways in which clinical problems may be present in the elderly. Moreover, he formulates the problem and the response in a fashion somewhat different from that used by other physicians. The geriatrician is required to be more concerned about the social and environmental etiologies as well as sensitive to the wide variety of physiologic deficits that can lead to the elderly patient's inability to cope. It is not enough to identify the common problems of old age as, for example, confusion, incontinence, falls, and loss of mobility; one must go further to identify the underlying processes that account for these dysfunctional behaviors to appreciate how such dysfunction will affect the lives of the old, and to assist in developing compensatory mechanisms (Engel 1977).

The geriatrician's task is determined by the characteristics of the patients he or she treats. The elderly as a group represent those with a higher prevalence of chronic illness, but despite these illnesses most are quite functional. The geriatrician's job is thus to facilitate that functioning by skillful intervention when appropriate and by knowledgeable nonintervention when the dangers of iatrogenic dysfunction outweigh any possible benefits.

The clinical decision-making paradigm, fundamental to the practice of good medicine, is tested in the extreme in the practice of geriatrics. The elderly patient may be thought of as an organism in delicate equilibrium with limited reserve capacities to withstand any external stress. Clinical experiences suggest that the factor that most sharply distinguishes the geriatric patient from other adult patients is just this reaction to stress. Baseline values in elderly patients are frequently within normal limits; it is only when some extra demand (such as an infection, an increased workload, or a drug side effect) is made that the lack of an adequate response reveals deficient reserves. Moreover, the same principle that applies to glucose intolerance applies to other dimensions of social, economic, and psychological activity as well. The loss of a spouse, the fracture of a hip, or an increase in rent may set in motion a chain of events leading to disastrous consequences for the patient.

The geriatrician must be able to deal with problem complexes involving several systems at once and with complex problems including unusual presentations of illness and limited resources to cope with them. Effective practice within this context requires skills and tools to disentangle such problems and sufficient expertise to identify both the probable and the possible. Particularly in view of the breadth of the domains to be covered, we have taken almost for granted the concept that geriatric care will involve teams of professionals. The geriatrician must be skilled in the mobilization and coordination of such resources. The team must be able to communicate in a common language and to show common goals. There must be a mechanism for recording these goals and for ascertaining progress toward them.

Medicine in general has been slow to emphasize prognosis. Although diagnosis implies some level of expected course for the patient, rarely are these expectations clearly articulated and almost never are they recorded. Because geriatrics deals with persons who are both compromised in their capacity to respond to stress and multiply afflicted by chronic disease, the need to think in terms of achievable benefit and avoidable dysfunction is all the greater. The geriatrician must be capable of practicing a highly skilled version of primary care in which he or she neither too readily dismisses a complaint as merely the inevitable consequence of aging nor overzealously pursues a condition for which there may be no useful remedy.

The traditional taxonomy of medicine must be augmented in geriatric practice to include paradigms that look beyond the usual descriptors of disease processes to emphasize the effects of illness on function. The geriatrician requires a set of measures that will allow him to ascertain the functional abilities of his patients to follow the course of change produced by treatment. These measures should cover the gamut of domains critical to the autonomous functioning of the elderly patient. In time, such measures will form the basis for appropriate clinical research to predict more accurately the kinds of results one might reasonably expect from multimodal treatments.

Because aged people are more likely to have chronic illness and are at greater risk of having more than one illness, their illnesses are more likely to be associated with or lead to disabilities. Neuromuscular difficulties may lead to disabilities in daily functions such as bathing, dressing, and walking. Weakness and decreased physical and mental tolerance to stress are more apt to cause geographic confinement and narrowed social interaction. In the presence of increased dependence on others (which is fostered by disability), there is often a paradoxical decrease in the number of able friends and family.

Along with isolation, ill and uncomfortable aging people are more vulnerable to desolation at times of personal crises such as the death of a spouse, geographic relocation, and change in social role. Socioeconomic productivity decreases, and financial resources may be depleted. Educational resources of those who are aged and ill are likely to become obsolete, and mental functioning slows. For those involved, there is an increased likelihood of such outcomes as deteriorating function and shorter life span. Dependency has serious consequences for the person, the family, and the community.

The mix of providers who care for the chronically ill aged and the interrelationships of such providers are different from those for acute-care providers. The structure and goals of services are different. The continuing cost of care increases the impact of decreasing socioeconomic productivity. Homemaking, medical, and income services are more likely to be needed for long periods of time. As a result, long-term care for the aged requires a unique system of services that integrates basic living supports and multidisciplinary elements of service. We are impressed with the fact that long-term care is both a treatment situation and a living situation. It encompasses institutional care and organized services that enable persons to remain at home with informal supportive aid from relatives or friends. It encompasses health care, supportive services, and the environments in which those with chronic conditions and disabilities live.

In view of the unique aspects of such care, those who care for the aged who are ill must have special knowledge and skills in order to assess the problems of the patient and the environment, define appropriate goals, and put a service plan into effect. The service plan generally requires bridged and coordinated services through shared information, where we define coordination as integrated decisions and actions in relation to particular professional goals. In addition, the service process is not an inflexible set of actions that follows a single set of goals. It is, rather, a dynamic process of changing goals and decisions, where the changes are based on feedback of information about improvement or lack of improvement and about the forces related to improvement or its absence.

The needs and demands of the chronically impaired aged can be expressed in physical, psychological, social, and environmental terms. Service decisions aim to improve our effectiveness with regard to outcomes of health maintenance, illness intervention, and the quality of life—at certain costs. In the absence of cure, outcome goals are formulated in such terms as restoration of function to the best possible level of partial dependence and dignity and its maintenance at that level. This framework establishes certain requirements for the type of information that we should include in our assessments of clients or patients. The information should be multidimensional, including physical, psychological, social, and economic descriptors. It should be objective, reliable, and amenable to systematic collection. It should be valid or meaningful and, in particular, should have demonstrated utility or relevance. For example, it should have demonstrated use in predicting resource needs or in describing improvement and deterioration of patients over time.

Long-term-care classification systems increasingly characterize the aged according to physical, psychological, social, and economic function. Measures of function are indicators of the existence, stage, and impact or outcome of chronic conditions; thus they become useful indicators of severity. Measures of function also offer a conceptual basis for defining homogeneous groupings in large population.

The geriatrician is often called on to assume responsibility for the elderly patient at the point when the constellation of health and related problems endangers the individual's ability to cope. Whether prompted by an acute event (such as a fall or an illness) or by a social circumstance, (such as the loss of a spouse), a final common pathway is decompensation. Geriatric practice reflects this situation by crossing the geographic boundaries of care to include assessment, rehabilitation, continuing care in the community, and long-term care in institutions.

The geriatrician should thus possess the requisite skills, attitudes, and knowledge to intervene in a manner that will foster the patient's ability to respond to the deterioration attributable to aging, the end results of accumulated illness, social dependency, and even the possibility of iatrogenic disability. The threat of iatrogenic illness is very real to the elderly patient. As the IOM report notes, these individuals are frequently exposed to surgical procedures and drugs. Both of these therapies can produce side effects that result in added disability. At a somewhat more subtle level, the elderly patient may suffer from another form of iatrogenic illness. The misapplication of diagnostic labels may result in a patient's being treated as more disabled than is the case. It is common to see patients condemned to nursing homes without an adequate search for treatable problems, and perhaps no label is as pernicious and as self-fulfilling as "senility."

Management skills are central to the repertoire of the geriatrician. Pfeiffer (1977) echoes the sentiments of many commentators on geriatrics in noting that

> The most important clinical service offered . . . is not a specific therapeutic intervention but rather the coordination effort of all services required by an individual while continuing contact is maintained with the individual.

Pollak (1979) has highlighted the reasons for the limitations of contemporary physician practice in this regard:

> . . . they are not challenged by the maintenance (rather than cure) objectives of such care; they often are uncomfortable or impatient with the heavy family and patient involvement that should enter long-term care decisions; they are often unfamiliar with the relevant networks of providers; and they are often pressed by matters that are or seem more urgent than the placing or counseling of someone whose medical condition is relatively stable.

The geriatrician will often find himself at the head of an interdisciplinary team composed of the variety of health workers needed to respond to the physical, social, and mental problems of the elderly. The geriatrician requires the skills to coordinate care in a variety of settings from home to acute hospital, nursing home to day hospital, clinic to day center. He must be able to prescribe drugs as well as services. He must be aware of the dangers of overtreatment and sensitive to those of overdiagnosis. Finally, in addition to collaborating with the multidisciplinary geriatric team, he is perhaps the sole member of that team who can interact appropriately with medical and surgical subspecialists such as urologists, orthopedists, or cardiologists so that medical and surgical strategies can be based on combined expertise.

The contribution of the geriatrician is well reflected in the achievements of the geriatric-evaluation unit (GEU). Patients destined for institutional long-term care placement have often been reassessed and rehabilitated. The GEU at the Little Rock, Arkansas, Veterans' Administration Medical Center reports that almost 75 percent of the GEU's patients have been returned to their homes. Preliminary data from the GEU indicate that an average of 3.39 new treatable problems were uncovered by GEU staff in the course of this assessment of each patient admitted to the unit directly upon discharge from the acute ward of a teaching hospital (personal communication from Owen Beard, M.D.).

A growing body of data has become available on the value of careful assessment of the elderly, particularly at the point when nursing-home care is being considered. Williams and his colleagues (1973) performed a comprehensive medical, nursing, and social evaluation on 315 patients referred for placement in nursing homes. As a result of the assessment, 23 percent were recommended to remain at home and only 35 percent were sent to a nursing home. Brocklehurst and his colleagues (1978) have demonstrated the ability of careful assessment to uncover treatable problems. Among 100 patients destined for institutionalization in an old-age home, thorough assessment uncovered 137 treatable physical disorders. As a result of the assessment, 32 patients were judged to be more appropriately placed in an alternative form of care.

In many ways the GEU may become as established a part of the hospital,s repertoire as the coronary-care unit. Such a development would serve to solidify the role of the geriatrician within the mainstream of medicine. As the demand for GEUs grows, so too will the need for geriatricians to direct and staff them.

Assessment units need not be hospital based. Several models of effective programs demonstrate how a comprehensive assessment of elderly patients can be used as a basis for planning long-term care. The emphasis is often on identifying modes of care other than nursing homes. The OARS programs at Duke University (Duke 1978), the TRIAGE project in Connecticut, and the ACCESS program in New York (U.S. Comptroller General 1979) all suggest that this approach is both feasible and effective. Although data are scant because of the newness of the projects, preliminary results are very encouraging. For example, ACCESS has been able to assist 89 percent of the Medicaid patients living in the community and 37 percent of the patients referred to nursing homes at the time of hospital discharge to return home (U.S. Comptroller General 1979).

In summary, although we take no position on the issue of whether geriatrics should be a specialty, we have come to accept the fact that a body of knowledge and a set of skills do exist and that they must be mastered in order to provide effective medical attention to the aged. We recognize that a well-trained internist could conceivably take on the role of geriatrician, but in so doing he would be obliged to alter some practice habits and to acquire additional knowledge. The motivated physician seeking to become a geriatrician might have to unlearn a number of ways of doing things. Perhaps most fundamentally, he may have to overcome his preoccupation with technology (Eisdorfer 1979). The hospital-trained, procedure-oriented, contemporary graduate may encounter some difficulty in making the transition to the more personalized, environmentally sensitive mode of practice needed in geriatrics. In part, the practice of geriatrics calls for rethinking one's approach to the problems faced by the aged. To the extent that we limit our discussion of the aged to those over age 75, the problems most commonly faced are a result of chronic illness and its sequelae.

Roles for the Geriatrician

The deficiencies in contemporary care of the elderly are attributable less to quantitative than to qualitative shortfalls. As we will show in chapter 4, the elderly do not receive substantially fewer services (even adjusted for need) than do younger persons. Rather, the difficulties arise because the quality of those services is inadequate. The elderly are medicine's lonely crowd.

Unfortunately, geriatrics may be viewed as predominantly nursing-home care (Libow 1978). We view this emphasis as unduly limiting the practice of the geriatrician in both scope and potential for effecting positive change in patient status. The bulk of care to persons aged 65 and older is given outside the nursing home. A simple calculation shows that less than 10 percent of the physician visits to this age group are to nursing-home patients.[1] Even if the geriatrician were to focus his attention on the more seriously ill patients, the nursing home is disproportionately represented in Libow's projections. Moreover, it may be an unwise strategy to create a career path that is so firmly linked to an institution generally shunned by other physicians. Although the nursing home is in desperate need of improvement and upgrading, this end may be better served by developing a cadre of physicians better trained to serve the elderly in general.

The present burden of geriatric care rests primarily on the shoulders of primary-care providers and is likely to remain there for the foreseeable future. This report builds on the recommendations of the IOM report in seeking ways in which some of that responsibility might be shared. In addressing this question, we have preferred to focus on roles that geriatricians might play, leaving aside the important and politically charged question of whether there should be a separate specialty. Four prototypes of geriatric activity can be easily identified along a spectrum; in order of presentation, each involves increasing numbers of geriatric medical manpower.

1. The most familiar and least disruptive scenario is one in which we change little or nothing. Those physicians who wish (or are persuaded) to care for the elderly continue to do so. A corollary aspect of the status quo is that little care is delegated to nonphysicians.
2. A second approach would concentrate on developing a cadre of geriatricians whose work would be limited to academic pursuits. We have already shown that the absolute and relative growth of the geriatric population has produced a consensus that commensurate changes in the medical-school curriculum are needed to prepare tomorrow's doctors to care for a growing number of elderly patients. This educational effort will surely require trained faculty to teach the future primary-care providers.

On this issue, we differ with the recommendations of the IOM. It does not appear feasible to conscript the necessary academic geriatric faculty from existing faculty in internal medicine and related disciplines. We cannot and should not attempt to make do with "instant geriatricians." The knowledge base, the practice skills, and the emphases embodied in a geriatrician are not so readily transferable. Although such temporary measures may be the only feasible response to the immediate crisis, it is misleading to confuse acts of necessity with planned goals.

Even a limited effort to produce academic geriatricians, however, has a direct effect on practice. A reasonable expectation is that as much as 25 percent of an academic geriatrician's time will be spent in patient care, both to maintain his skills and to develop training sites. Moreover, experience in preparing academic physicians in other subareas of internal medicine indicates that there is invariably a group of individuals trained in such programs who forsake their academic goals and choose to enter practice (Scheele and Kitzes 1969). A cohort of trained geriatric practitioners can thus be anticipated as a byproduct of the attempt to fill the academic near vacuum.

3. The geriatrician's clinical role could extend beyond the academic walls but be limited to that of the true specialist seeing patients only on referral and providing consultation to other providers about patient-management problems. Such a model closely resembles the mode of practice of the British geriatric specialist and would allow for practice in a variety of settings but not for the provision of primary care.

4. Finally, the geriatrician would provide a substantial proportion of the primary care for the elderly in addition to filling the specialist role, more akin to what Fry (1970) has termed "specialoid" practice. The rate of assuming primary-care responsibilities might be timed to approximate the growth of the elderly segment of the population as as to minimize any disruption to those already providing care to the elderly. Primary care from geriatricians would thus be directed at the additional cohorts of the elderly entering the appropriate age range.

Forecasts of physician manpower predict substantial increases in the number of doctors per capita. Our projections of manpower do not call for new or additional physicians to be trained beyond those already planned. Rather we seek to explore ways in which that pool of physicians might be redistributed to offer better care to the elderly.

Although we have suggested that the four models discussed here call for a redistribution of physician effort, with no demands for larger numbers of physicians to be trained, other modes of redistribution should be considered as well. Much of the care burden could be shared through delegation to providers such as the nurse practitioner and the physician's assistant or to those more prepared to manage social and mental problems (that is, social workers). As is the case in primary care (including primary care of the elderly), the possible extent of delegation is very large in concept. Several different patterns of this delegation are worthy of examination, ranging from a very conservative position to a much more liberal one; these patterns are described in chapter 5. Within this spectrum, we see the basic model of the geriatrician as the manager of a care team or teams.

Choices of Roles

From the array of models just presented, we favor those that anticipate the geriatrician in both the academic and practicing roles. We would further predict that the geriatrician will have to provide at least some first-contact care rather than relying solely on referrals from other-care physicians. We anticipate that the geriatrician's primary-care caseload will derive from two sources. He will be sought out directly by elderly patients, and he will assume the responsibility for ongoing care of a portion of those patients initially referred by other physicians. Our projected role for the geriatrician thus falls between those outlined as prototypes 3 and 4 in the preceding list; those descriptions, in turn, serve as useful boundaries for our estimates of geriatric-manpower needs. As will be shown in chapter 5, even modest estimations would suggest that some degree of delegation to nonphysician providers will be necessary; we argue that it may be very desirable as well.

    A number of factors have persuaded us that geriatrics should and will include practice as well as teaching.

    1. A substantial portion of geriatric care is related to problems of geropsychiatry, especially dementia and depression, occurring in patients having a considerable burden of physical illness as well. Geropsychiatrists are not readily available; primary-care physicians lack the psychiatric skills; and psychiatrists lack the medical skills to diagnose and manage these cases. The geriatrician is the logical choice.

    2. The unsatisfactory quality of care currently witnessed in the medical management of the elderly will not be greatly improved if geriatrics is confined to the academic teaching hospital. The improvement of care requires the leadership and active presence of geriatricians in the community as well as in the academic centers.

    3. Precedents strongly suggest that geriatrics cannot be confined to the academic center. In this regard, we take issue with the IOM report wherein it is argued that geriatrics, like genetics, can serve its full function confined to an academic milieu. The geriatrician, as previously outlined, is the logical consultant for the infirm elderly with complex medical and psychosocial

problems. Such patients are exceedingly common throughout the community; by no means are they confined to academic medical centers. In fact, they are apt to be underrepresented there. This is very different from the situation in genetics, where the geneticist has an important function in the teaching setting but is clearly not in demand as a consultant in the community.

Geriatrics is far more analogous to infectious disease than to geriatrics. Infectious disease is a subspecialty of internal medicine that at first prospered only in the academic medical centers but soon expanded into the community as its consultative contribution to patient care became appreciated. Like geriatrics, its field cuts across all the organ-specific subspecialties of internal medicine; this has neither hampered its growth nor created major territorial conflicts. When the infectious problem dominates the clinical picture or poses issues too complex for the generalist, the internist with an organ-system subspecialty, or the nonmedical specialist to handle confidently, then the infectious-disease specialist is called. The infectious-disease specialist uses other specialists and subspecialists as consultants for patients with major problems in the various systems. Correspondingly, the geriatrician will be consulted when the complexity of multisystem medical problems and psychosocial issues is overwhelming to the physician in charge. On the other hand, the geriatrician will consult with other types of physicians when the problems in a particular organ system or discipline require it.

4. Geriatric medicine goes beyond consultative functions to encompass a primary-care role as well. Geriatric medicine is analogous to the organ-system subspecialties of internal medicine (Aiken et al. 1979). In these subspecialties, a very important percentage of physicians' time is spent delivering primary care to patients whose predominant problem is usually, but not always, in their subspecialty area. Similarly, the geriatrician will undoubtedly assume a primary-care responsibility (with full agreement of all concerned) for many patients who will have first seen him or her as a consultant. This should and will happen where continuing care is necessary and where the previous primary physician no longer feels competent to deal with the range of uniquely geriatric problems afflicting the patient.

5. Practicing geriatricians are almost a natural consequence of any substantial effort to train a cadre of academics. Some graduates, perhaps as many as half, will pursue practicing careers in the community. We term this phenomenon the "spillover" effect.

6. There is a clearly identifiable need for geriatricians in institutions and agencies that are not academic, such as larger skilled-nursing facilities, larger residential complexes, and agencies for home-based long-term care. It is impossible for full-time academicians to provide the necessary leadership and day-to-day medical care for these institutions and agencies.

7. Public demand for geriatric services will stimulate a response among physicians regardless of what is done formally. The issue is how to improve and strengthen that response. Although small in number, a cadre of geriatricians now exists, as described in chapter 2. They are poorly trained for the task, and most have drifted into it from other specialties. If they are going to exist, why not have them well prepared?

Note

1. The 23 million elderly average 5.9 (or 6.8, depending on recall period) physician visits annually. If we assume that the 989,000 elderly nursing-home residents are seen monthly (an overestimate), the ratio is $(989,000 \times 12) \div (23,000,000 \times 5.9) = 0.087$. Alternatively, one can look ahead to the data in appendix B, table B-5, where the proportion of nursing-home visits to total medical physician visits is 0.02 for those 65 to 74 years old and 0.9 for those over 75.

4

The Need for Academic Geriatricians

For purposes of estimating the need for geriatricians now and in the future, we address two major roles, those of the academic geriatrician and the practicing geriatrician. This chapter deals with estimates of the former.

It is necessary to estimate in some way the number of geriatric medical faculty required in the United States to carry out the following missions:

1. To introduce geriatric material into the undergraduate medical and other health-professional curricula.
2. To develop geriatric-medical segments of internal-medicine and family-practice residency programs.
3. To conduct fellowship training of future geriatric-medicine faculty and specialists and to participate in similar fellowships for geropsychiatrists.
4. To contribute to the education of geriatric nurse practitioners and physician's assistants.
5. To engage in research in gerontology or geriatrics.
6. To provide a segment of patient care for elderly persons, usually referred patients with very complex problems.

We shall assume that approximately 25 percent of faculty members' professional effort is devoted to patient care and the remaining 75 percent to the other five academic functions listed. The number of geriatric faculty required cannot be determined on the basis of units of patient-care services needed, as we shall do for the practicing geriatric specialist. Rather, we must estimate the teaching "loads" (items 1 through 4) and calculate manpower need from these. Then the contribution to patient care provided by this number of geriatric medical academicians can be subtracted from the units of service that must be provided by nonacademic geriatric specialists.

The academic need is distributed among medical schools, "primary" teaching hospitals, and other teaching hospitals. It is driven primarily by the educational requirements of medical students, residents in internal medicine and family practice, and geriatric fellows. Demands of lesser magnitude are placed by nursing students and geropsychiatry residents; these will be ignored in our estimates. The Institute of Medicine (IOM) report has recommended that each medical school mount a teaching program in

47

geriatric medicine. We concur. It also states, however, that the geriatric faculty needed are, for the most part, already available at the academic center. With this, we do not agree. It is our belief that, although converted internists, family physicians, and others may fill the vacuum at the outset, the midterm and longer development of academic geriatric medicine requires a cadre of new, authentic, trained-for-the-purpose geriatricians. If they are to stand as effective role models, these academic geriatricians must be familiar with the content of geriatrics and with its emphasis on the management of patients (see the previous chapter). Such geriatricians will be well versed in measurement in the elderly; they will be able to distinguish small but important increments of change in the status of their patients. Their research interests will include problems affecting the delivery of better care to the elderly, as well as biomedical investigations into the diseases that account for so much of the disability among the elderly. (This book contains separate chapters on measurement and research, where these points are further elaborated.)

Although we cannot prove this contention, no other specialty or subspecialty has ever staffed its faculty positions by borrowed faculty any longer than was required to produce products of its own training program. Hence, as we project needs for 1990, we must postulate that the great majority of geriatric-medical faculty will have received formal training, and that by 2010 and 2030 all will have been so educated. Therefore, faculty needs would be supplied by geriatric specialists rather than being interchangeable with medical subspecialists and primary-care physicians, as would be inferred from the recommendation of the IOM report.

The Geriatric Program

We make the assumption that a medical school's geriatric program should have at least two full-time faculty members; one-person teaching units are not viable for more than a short time. Considering the variation in the size of medical schools, their programs, and their resources for faculty support, we estimate that a conservative average would be three full-time geriatric-medical faculty members per medical school, a total of 372. These three will handle the undergraduate medical curriculum, undergraduate nursing education (where needed), part of the geriatric components of the medical and family-practice residencies at the "primary" university teaching hospital, and any geriatric fellowship program located there. It cannot be assumed that any teaching time will be left to cover the needs of affiliated and nonaffiliated teaching hospitals. Additional faculty are therefore needed.

To define the latter requirement accurately is difficult, but we can make reasonable lower-bound and upper-bound estimates. For the upper-bound estimate, we ignore program size and assume that all residencies in internal medicine and family practice will eventually require geriatric faculty. At this future time, we estimate a need for an average of 2.0 faculty members for each internal-medicine residency and 1.5 for each family-practice residency. (It should be emphasized that these figures are offered as approximate means, not as either ceilings or floors.) Where both residency programs exist in a hospital, we assume an economy of scale of 1 faculty member, for a total of 2.5. In the principal university hospital, we assume that the core medical-school faculty can simultaneously handle half of the teaching needs of the residency programs. Thus we must add only 1 faculty member if an internal-medicine residency is offered there, 0.75 if a family-practice residency is offered, but not further economy-of-scale factor if both are offered.

For the lower-bound estimate, we assume that the size of training programs is not going to change greatly and that smaller programs will not be able to add geriatric-medicine specialists to their faculty. Specifically, small internal-medicine programs with 0 to 9 full-time faculty and 0 to 29 residents (including all three years) are assigned no such faculty; those of medium size with 10 to 19 faculty and/or 30 to 49 residents are assigned 1.0; and those of larger size with 20 or more faculty and/or 50 or more residents are assigned 2.0. If 20 or more faculty are present with 0 to 29 residents, or if 0 to 9 faculty coincide with 50 or more residents, 1.0 teacher of geriatrics is assigned. Among family-practice programs, which tend to run smaller than internal-medicine residencies, no faculty in geriatrics are assigned to small programs with 0 to 3 faculty and 0 to 17 residents. For medium-sized programs with 4 to 6 faculty and/or 18 to 29 residents, an average of 0.75 faculty member is assigned; for large programs with 7 or more faculty and/or 30 or more residents, 1.5 faculty members are assigned. If 7 or more faculty are present with 0 to 17 residents, or if 0 to 3 faculty coincide with 30 or more residents, the intermediate level of 0.75 faculty member is assigned. As in the case of the upper-bound estimates, assignments are lowered to account for economy of utilization of faculty when a family-practice and an internal-medicine program coexist in a teaching hospital. One-half is subtracted if one program is large and the other is large or medium in size; 0.25 faculty member is subtracted if both programs are medium sized. Finally, calculated faculty requirements were halved for residency programs in the primary university teaching hospitals, but no further subtraction was introduced for having both internal-medicine and family-practice programs in such a hospital.

Using data provided by the National Study of Internal Medicine Manpower and the *Guide to Family Practice Residency Programs* published by the American Academy of Family Physicians and the American Medical

Student Association (1979), we determined that there were, in early 1979, 456 residency programs in internal medicine, of which 128 coexisted with a family-practice residency in the hospital and 328 did not. There were 358 family-practice residencies, of which 230 were in hospitals without internal-medicine programs. Calculation of upper-bound estimates according to the decision rules outlined in the preceding paragraphs yielded a figure of 1,231 faculty members in geriatric medicine for supervision of residency programs. Combined with the estimate of 372 for medical schools (124 schools × 3 faculty per school), this results in an upper-bound estimate of 1,603, which we have rounded to 1,600. The lower-bound estimate, similarly enumerated, was 517 for residency programs and 889 overall. The latter figure was rounded to 900 for the purposes of this book.

The reader should appreciate that the projections offered are static. For purposes of these estimates, we have assumed that the complement of academic geriatricians will be instantaneously available and will remain at the same level through 2030. No effort has been made to describe a phasing-in process (although we argue in chapter 8 that this mode is desirable). Nor do we allow for expansion in the number of schools to be staffed or in the size of faculties. However, this acknowledged artificiality should not substantially compromise the usefulness of the estimates and their appro-priateness to the relatively crude level of available data.

Spillover Effect

Having estimated the number of faculty needed to staff necessary positions in medical schools and teaching hospitals, we now need to look at the train-ing side of the equation. Recognizing that we take off from a standing start, we could not hope to reach the goals until 1990, which is ten years away. As detailed in chapter 2, by July 1, 1980, there will be a potential capacity for approximately 42 new fellows to enter fellowship training in geriatric medicine annually; but we must predict that, based on experience to date, less than three-fourths of these positions will be filled. Previous data from National Institutes of Health (NIH) training programs in gastroenterology (Scheele and Kitzes 1969) indicate that the yield of full-time academicians is proportionate to the number of years of training: highest (over 60 percent) for three-year trainees, and rather low (less than 20 percent, with a major emphasis on research) for those with only one year of training. Thus we propose, for geriatric medicine, two years of training for 75 percent of fellows and three years for 25 percent; our recommendation would be for even more three-year trainees, but we doubt that sufficient funding will be available. Thus in 1982 up to 32 trained geriatricians with two years of training will enter the job market. In 1983 and each year thereafter, up to 42 will complete training (32 with two years of training and 10 with three years). Assuming that all fellowships will be filled from 1981-1982 on, there will be approximately 400 graduates, including those finishing in June 1990.

The actual number could be larger if additional training programs are developed and funded between 1980 and 1988. This is difficult to estimate. It is unlikely that the Veterans Administration will increase its fellowship support very much. If additional Geriatric Research, Education, and Clinical Centers (GRECCs) are funded and launched, it is possible that as many as fifteen fellowship programs could develop, an increase of four. In the private sector, the only sizable additional support that can be visualized would be from the National Institute on Aging (NIA). Meanwhile, potential sites in universities are scarce because of a "chicken-and-egg" phenomenon; there are too few faculty at most schools to provide the critical mass needed to develop an advanced preacademic training program.

One serious flaw runs through this entire discussion. The previously mentioned Scheele-Kitzes study (1969), as well as a wide sampling of opinions of NIH and Association of American Medical Colleges (AAMC) administrators, indicates that between 40 and 50 percent of NIH trainees end up in full-time academic positions. Some administrators made considerably lower estimates; but those who are now analyzing the recent version of the NIH training grant, the National Research Service Award (Institutional), believe that the yield from 1975 on is apt to be higher, although data are not yet available. The "payback" provision is thought by many to be more effective than various screening methods in identifying those with the most enduring motivation for academic careers. It seems unlikely, however, that any training program demanding three years of intensive effort after a three-year core residency will yield more than 60 percent who will resist the attractions of private practice.

This upper-bound figure, then, needs to be applied back to our manpower estimates for academicians. In order to harvest the 900 geriatric clinician-teacher-researchers needed for academic posts, we must train 1,500 fellows. Obviously, this is a distant target because we have already suggested that attainable numbers will not exceed 33 percent of this number by 1990. The other corollary of this concept of a certain obligatory fraction of "recidivism" is that a significant number of geriatric specialists with training suitable for a consultant role in the community will be produced pari passu with any training program designed to produce academicians. In meeting or approaching the faculty needs, we will automatically create at least a small cadre of practicing geriatric specialists. This will become the corps of a new specialty whether we seek it or not.

5 Estimating Need for Practicing Geriatricians

As noted earlier, our projections of geriatric-medical manpower are dual estimates: those geriatricians needed to fill academic roles and those available for direct patient care. The former have been described in the preceding chapter. This chapter summarizes the strategy used to estimate the need for the latter. These techniques are then applied to produce boundary estimates for the four levels of geriatric activity already noted. Under this model, geriatric manpower is assumed to come from some redistribution of existing, or potentially available but unused, manpower. Here again, however, the distinction is not crucial for the purposes of the present model (although critics will correctly point out the cost implications if geriatricians are simply laid on top of an already well-stocked manpower supply).

In this study, our estimate of the number of physicians needed to care for the elderly population is based on a series of calculations. The number of physicians needed to provide current levels of service in a given year is the sum of the number needed for each age group (65 to 74 and over 75). That, in turn, is the product of the number of persons in each age group in the year at issue and the number of units of service per person (determined from user-based or provider-based data). The total units are then divided by physician productivity, that is, the number of units of service that can be provided per year by one physician, to yield the number of full-time-equivalent (FTE) physicians needed. Because the available data deal with hospital and nonhospital services separately, we calculate physician FTE requirements separately for these two types of services and then add them together. We next divide the required services among various types of physician and nonphysician health-care providers. Each pattern of division calls for a corresponding change in the productivity factors used in the equation. Finally, figures based on "need" may be substituted (when available) for the demand-based figures used here, and the rest of the equation remains unchanged. We have translated "need" into a concept of "improved care." The level of improved care was derived from a regression equation of National Health Interview Survey data to estimate the extent of underutilization by the elderly if correlations were made for their health status and socioeconomic status. To this we added the increased utilization obtained if the encounter time for the elderly was equal to that for younter cohorts. The result was a multiplied constant of 1.26 for the total population aged 65 and older and of 1.28 if only those over age 75 were addressed. Readers interested in the details of our methodological strategies and assumptions should refer to appendix B.

Personnel Configurations

An important variable in the equation for estimating manpower demand is the partition of care among different types of physicians and nonphysicians. In chapter 3, we described four alternative levels of geriatrician involvement in the care of the elderly, ranging from a minimal role (the status quo) to a very extensive role (in academic medical centers, in consultative practice, and in primary care). With each increment in the participation by the geriatricians, the fraction of care of the elderly delivered by medical subspecialists and primary-care physicians must decline. To develop our boundary estimates, we have translated these qualitative descriptions into representative percentage of effort (table 5-1). This quantification is admittedly arbitrary and is intended to provide a gross estimate of the distribution of workload for each assumed pattern of care.

Because team care has been widely advocated as a means of achieving more and better geriatric care, we have then proposed three possible patterns of shared workload between the geriatric specialist or the primary-care physician and geriatric nurse practitioners (GNPs), or physician's assistants (PAs), or social workers (SWs) (table 5-2). The minimum level of

Table 5-1
Partition (Percentage) of Effort of Health-Care Personnel in the Care of the Elderly: Effect of Training Programs Aimed at Different Geriatrician Roles

Type of Training	Nonhospital Care[a]			Hospital Care		
	GS	MSS	PCP	GS	MSS	PCP
1. Status quo	1	14	85	1	19	80
2. Training geriatricians for academic positions only	—	—	—	—	—	—
3. Training geriatricians for academic positions and as consultants in practice	25	10	65	20	15	65
4. Training geriatricians for academic positions, as consultants, and as primary-care physicians	40	10	50	30	15	55

Note: GS = geriatric specialist; MSS = medical subspecialist (cardiologist, gastroenterologist, and so on); PCP = primary-care physician (internist, family physician, general practitioner).
[a] Includes ambulatory care, nursing-home care, and common alternatives to nursing-home care.

Table 5-2
Partition (Percentage) of Effort of Health-Care Personnel in the Care of the Elderly: Delegation of Physician Functions to Nonphysicians

Level of Delegation	Nonhospital Care [a]			Hospital Care		
	MD [b]	PA/GNP	SW	MD	PA/GNP	SW
Minimal (status quo)	95	3	2	100	0	0
Moderate	65	25	10	90	10	0
Maximal	40	40	20	80	20	0

Note: PA/GNP = physician assistant or geriatric nurse practitioner; SW = social worker.
[a] Includes ambulatory care, outpatient, hospital, nursing-home care, and common alternatives to nursing-home care.
[b] Only GS and PCP are assumed to delegate. MD refers only to nonsurgical physicians.

delegation corresponds roughly to the present situation. The medium and maximum extents of delegation are chosen to represent points on a spectrum without any specific model in mind. Experience to date with PAs and GNPs suggests that no specific delegation patterns of certain types of patients over others is likely to occur. Except for the extent to which the supervising physician sees the difficult cases of the PAs or GNPs, the practice profiles of the PAs and the GNPs appear very similar to that of the supervising physician. Medical suspecialists have not been expected to delegate part of their work to these nonphysicians. To the extent that the subspecialists may delegate, some of the physician model calls for delegation of subspecialty work to the other physician categories.

For the most part, the academic and practice parts of the geriatric-manpower pool can be estimated separately and simply combined at will. One area of possible interface is attributable to the inefficiency of the production of academic physicians. As has been noted, we are only about 50-percent efficient in training physicians for academic careers; about half of those so trained are likely to enter practice instead. Therefore, any estimate of academic-training investments will have some spillover effect on the number of available practitioners. On the other hand, those in academic clinical medicine often spend a portion of their time—perhaps as much as a quarter of it—in direct care of patients. This pool of services should be taken into account.

Personnel Need

As we have noted, our estimates of manpower needs are based on current utilization adjusted for projected demographic changes and the extent to which additional needs could be met. We now introduce one additional variable into the projections. We could consider geriatricians to be responsible for varying portions of the care of those aged 65 and older; alternatively, we could assume that efforts of geriatricians will primarily concentrate on patients aged 75 and older, the group likely to contain more of the frail elderly.

Table 5-3 presents a point of departure, represented by our estimates of the total number of physician visits (both hospital and nonhospital) that we anticipate for persons in this age group for the years of interest. From 1977 to 2030, the anticipated use of medical services for those aged 65 and older will more than double; for those aged 75 and older, the use will almost triple.

When these utilization estimates are combined with productivity data, we can translate them into manpower estimates (see appendix B). Ignoring for a moment the need for academic geriatricians, we can see in table 5-4 estimates of the number of physician personnel needed in 1977 and 2010, under three different modes of geriatric practice, to care for persons aged 65 and older. (The proportion of care provided by the geriatric specialist is shown in table 5-1.) Levels of geriatric manpower as high as 23,000 may be somewhat intimidating, especially noting that estimates of academic need and improved care are not included in table 5-4. Two basic recourses are available to reduce this potential burden: restriction of the target population (that is, focusing geriatric care on those aged 75 and older) and increased use of nonphysician providers. Table 5-5 shows the number of physician personnel that will be needed in 2010 to care for persons aged 75 and older under the same modes of practice as those shown in table 5-4. Only one-half as many geriatricians are required if the age range is narrowed.

The effects of two levels of delegation on physician manpower requirements to care for persons aged 65 and older in 2010 are shown in table 5-6. Moderate delegation would achieve a little more than a 20-percent reduction in the geriatric-physician manpower needed, whereas maximal delegation could achieve almost a 50-percent reduction. But maximal delegation implies the availability of large numbers of trained intermediate health professionals. For example, the maximal-delegation projection shown in table 5-6 calls for more than 20,000 GNPs or PAs. Used together, maximal delegation and restriction of the target population to those over age 75 could reduce the need for geriatric-physician manpower to only 30 percent of that indicated in table 5-4.

Having examined some of the ways in which individual aspects of the projection model may affect our estimates of personnel needed to provide geriatric-medical services, we can turn our attention to the various predictions of the need for geriatricians under a variety of situations. Tables 5-7 and 5-8 summarize these situations for levels based on current utilization

Table 5-3
Estimated Annual Physician Visits (Hospital and Nonhospital) for Persons 65 Years and Older, 1977-2030

	Visits per Year (millions)			
Age Group	1977	1990	2010	2030
65+	186.8	238.4	281.1	442.6
75+	83.7	114.1	143.6	220.6

Table 5-4
Number of Physician Personnel (in FTEs) Needed in 1977 and 2010 to Care for Persons 65 Years and Older at Current Utilization Levels

	Number of Physician Personnel Required					
	1977			2010		
Mode of Geriatric Practice	GS	MSS	PCP	GS	MSS	PCP
Status quo	432	730	22,772	655	1,109	34,453
Consultative	9,915	5,484	17,808	15,000	8,330	26,953
Primary care	15,509	5,484	14,214	23,452	8,330	21,527

Note: GS = geriatric specialist; MSS = medical subspecialist; PCP = primary-care physician (general internist, family physician, general practitioner).

Table 5-5
Number of Physicians (in FTEs) Needed in 2010 to Care for Persons 75 Years and Older at Current Utilization Levels

	Number of Physicians Required		
Mode of Geriatric Practice	Geriatric Specialist	Medical Subspecialist	Primary-Care Physician
Status quo	335	577	17,441
Consulative	7,587	4,357	13,688
Primary care	11,823	4,357	10,987

and improved care, respectively. These two tables give estimates of the total need for both practicing and academic geriatricians. Using the previously proposed assumption that 25 percent of the academicians' time will be used to provide direct geriatric care, we have summed the number of geriatricians

Table 5–6
Number of Physician and Nonphysician Personnel (in FTEs) Needed in 2010 to Care for Persons 65 Years and Older at Current Utilization Levels Under Two Levels of Delegation

Mode of Geriatric Practice	Number of Physician and Nonphysician Personnel Required									
	Moderate Delegation					Maximal Delegation				
	GS	MS	PCP	GNP/PA	SW	GS	MS	PCP	GNP/PA	SW
Status quo	520	1,109	26,914	11,622	3,766	391	1,109	19,852	19,479	7,532
Consultative	11,702	8,330	21,156	12,169	3,941	8,618	8,330	15,692	20,398	7,882
Primary care	18,205	8,330	17,026	12,169	3,941	13,329	8,330	12,739	20,398	7,882

Note: GS = geriatric specialist; MSS = medical subspecialist; PCP = primary-care physician (general internist, family physician, general physician); GNP/PA = geriatric nurse practitioner or physician's assistant; SW = social worker.

Table 5-7
**Number of Geriatricians (in FTEs) Needed to Care for Persons Aged 65 +
and 75 + Under Various Levels of Delegation and Modes of Practice, Based
on Current Utilization Levels**

Level of Delegation to Nonphysicians	Mode of Geriatric Practice	Number of Geriatricians Required			
		1977	1990	2010	2030
Minimal	Status quo				
	65 +	432	555	655	1,031
	75 +	195	266	335	515
	Academic				
	65 +	1,500[a]	1,500	1,500	1,500
	75 +	1,500	1,500	1,500	1,500
	+ Consultative[b]				
	65 +	10,590	13,402	15,675	24,297
	75 +	5,096	6,704	8,262	12,331
	+ Primary care[b]				
	65 +	16,184	20,579	24,127	37,612
	75 +	7,565	10,071	12,498	18,840
Moderate	Status quo				
	65 +	342	440	520	818
	75 +	158	215	271	416
	Academic				
	65 +	1,500	1,500	1,500	1,500
	75 +	1,500	1,500	1,500	1,500
	+ Consultative[b]				
	65 +	8,577	10,777	12,561	19,280
	75 +	4,368	5,644	6,881	10,111
	+ Primary care[b]				
	65 +	12,873	16,292	19,064	29,520
	75 +	6,300	8,278	10,195	15,202
Maximal	Status quo				
	65 +	257	331	391	615
	75 +	121	165	208	319
	Academic				
	65 +	1,500	1,500	1,500	1,500
	75 +	1,500	1,500	1,500	1,500
	+ Consultative[b]				
	65 +	6,661	8,285	9,608	14,550
	75 +	3,626	4,585	5,514	7,940
	+ Primary care[b.]				
	65 +	9,764	12,274	14,419	21,963
	75 +	5,053	6,531	7,962	11,702

[a] 1,500 geriatricians need to be trained to provide 900 academic geriatricians after allowing for spillover.

[b] These figures include 75 percent of the 900 academic geriatricians and 25 percent FTE (225) duplicate practice needs.

Table 5-8
Number of Geriatricians (in FTEs) Needed to Care for Persons Aged 65 + and 75 + Under Various Levels of Delegation and Modes of Practice, If Care Is Improved

Level of Delegation to Nonphysicians	Mode of Geriatric Practice	Number of Geriatricians Required			
		1977	1990	2010	2030
Minimal	Status quo				
	65 +	542	697	823	1,295
	75 +	250	340	428	658
	Academic				
	65 +	1,500[a]	1,500	1,500	1,500
	75 +	1,500	1,500	1,500	1,500
	+ Consultative[b]				
	65 +	13,160	16,718	19,606	30,475
	75 +	6,362	8,425	10,433	15,667
	+ Primary care[b]				
	65 +	20,223	25,790	30,306	47,321
	75 +	9,552	12,780	15,907	24,077
Moderate	Status quo				
	65 +	427	550	650	1,022
	75 +	200	273	343	527
	Academic				
	65 +	1,500	1,500	1,500	1,500
	75 +	1,500	1,500	1,500	1,500
	+ Consultative[b]				
	65 +	10,529	13,294	15,547	23,971
	75 +	5,333	6,960	8,537	12,655
	+ Primary care[b]				
	65 +	15,925	20,231	23,735	36,858
	75 +	7,808	10,335	12,783	19,179
Maximal	Status quo				
	65 +	318	410	485	763
	75 +	152	207	260	400
	Academic				
	65 +	1,500	1,500	1,500	1,500
	75 +	1,500	1,500	1,500	1,500
	+ Consultative[b]				
	65 +	8,050	10,079	11,737	17,893
	75 +	4,318	5,528	6,701	9,764
	+ Primary care[b]				
	65 +	11,926	15,065	17,630	27,164
	75 +	6,128	7,977	9,807	14,536

[a] 1,500 geriatricians need to be trained to provide 900 academic geriatricians after allowing for spillover.

[b] These figures include 75 percent of the 900 academic geriatricians and 25 percent FTE (225) duplicate practice needs.

needed for practice and 0.75 times the number needed to fill academic posts to reach the estimates identified as "and consultative" and "and primary care" in these tables. As indicated earlier, these tables point up the infeasibility of a purely academic model. Even if the goal were to produce only academic geriatricians, the spillover effect would provide 2 practitioners for every 3 academicians. Thus 1,500 geriatric trainees would be needed to yield 900 academicians, and these 900 would produce an average of 225 FTEs of service.

Tables 5-7 and 5-8 are organized to show several effects together. For each level of delegation, four modes of geriatric practice are examined. For each of these modes, estimates of need for geriatric FTEs are projected to serve a population of all those over age 65 and for only those over age 75. The result is a very wide range of estimates. At the lower extreme, in 1977 it would require 195 geriatricians to approximate the status quo if only those patients aged 75 and older were considered; but if one wanted to use geriatricians to deliver consultative services and a portion of the primary-care services to those aged 65 and older today (that is, 1977), and to provide for a cadre of academic geriatricians, then more than 16,000 might be required.

Although the assumptions on which these estimates depend could be challenged, it is useful to consider the order of magnitude that these projections suggest. Assuming little or no delegation to nonphysicians, more than 40,000 geriatricians would be needed to provide even 30 percent of "improved" care to those over age 65 by the year 2030. Hence, most geriatric-care services are likely to be provided by nongeriatricians. Some will argue that we will be hard pressed just to meet the academic needs.

Other Predictions of Geriatric Manpower

It is interesting to compare our projections of needed geriatric manpower with those of Libow (1978). In testimony before a congressional subcommittee, he estimated a need for approximately 8,000 to 10,000 geriatricians. His reasoning was based on the following role allocations for these geriatricians:

1-4 geriatricians for each teaching hospital	=	500-2,000
1-4 geriatricians for each medical school	=	121-484
1 geriatrician for each physician's-assistant and nurse-practitioner training program	=	93
1 geriatrician in each state health department	=	50
1 geriatrician in each retirement community	=	100
1 geriatrician in each skilled-nursing facility	=	7,000
Total		7,864-9,727

Libow then recommended a massive effort to establish a training program to meet the deficit in four years. Again this strategy differs from the one we will propose in chapter 7.

Others may feel that the numbers of geriatricians called for by one or another of the models offered are excessive. We would point out that the estimates are based on redistributed activities and can thus be used to assess the implications of other configurations as they are put forward. For example, were we to project on the basis of the course recommended in the Institute of Medicine report (1978), 1,500 trained geriatricians would suffice to meet both academic needs and, through spillover, the limited need for consultants. If we pursue the level of geriatric activity advocated in chapter 3 (assuming a moderate degree of delegation), we interpolate a need for approximately 8,000 geriatricians in 1990 (from table 5-8).

6

Projections of the Need for Geropsychiatrists

This chapter completes our estimates of the need for physician manpower to provide the full range of geriatric services. We have chosen to deal with the need for geropsychiatrists in a separate chapter because the data are derived from different sources and the productivity of psychiatric care seems quite different from the medical figures we have used previously.

Mental illness is perhaps the most difficult area in medicine for which to predict the need for care. Estimates of the prevalence and incidence of problems related to mental illness range widely. Nonetheless, there is general agreement that a substantial part of geriatric care both now and in the future will involve the treatment of mental illness in the elderly, including illness related to dementia and to more acute and chronic psychoses. Because of the difficulty in making clear statements about need, it seems most appropriate to look at several different approaches by which quantitative bounds might be put on the projected need for geropsychiatric services.

Estimates Based on Utilization

The first approach is based on two assumptions:

1. The utilization of geropsychiatric services in the future will be related to the present utilization of psychiatric services by individuals 65 years of age and older.
2. An additional need for geropsychiatric services will be created by the demand for geropsychiatrists in an academic role to train future geropsychiatrists, psychiatrists, geriatricians, and mental-health workers.

These assumptions anticipate that a substantial part of the treatment of mental illness among the elderly would be provided by psychiatrists other than geropsychiatrists. This approach is complementary to the approach taken to estimate geriatric-manpower requirements in the sense that physician visits for identified psychiatric problems had been omitted from those calculations. Thus, reintroducing the set of services at this point is a nonduplicative addition.

The USC/DRME data indicate that the average psychiatrist spends about 0.9 hour in patient care at the hospital per day and 3.2 hours of patient care in nonhospital activities. Of the hospital encounters, 13 percent are devoted to patients aged 65 and older; for the nonhospital encounters, the figure is 3.1 percent. The weighted average of combining these two yields a figure of 0.22 hour per day out of a total of 4.1 hours per day spent on patient care devoted to people 65 years and older; in other words, 5.3 percent of the total patient-care time is spent on the elderly. Multiplying this percentage by the 21,478 psychiatrists in the country (Goodman 1979), we identify a demand for 1,130 full-time equivalents (FTEs) in 1977. This figure can then be projected upward in the same manner as the geriatric-manpower projections, a calculation that yields the following FTE needs:

Year	Number of FTEs
1977	1,130
1990	1,440
2010	1,690
2030	2,660

These numbers represent the FTEs required to meet current utilization of psychiatric services by the elderly, adjusted for demographic projections.

To this figure we would then add the need for academic geropsychiatrists. One means of estimating this need is to assume that the academic geropsychiatrists will be used to train three classes of practitioners: future academic geropsychiatrists, psychiatrists who will treat the elderly, and geriatricians in both practice and academic settings. For purposes of this estimation, let us assume that there would be 15 national programs training academic geropsychiatrists (about twice the number currently available), that all psychiatric training programs would have geropsychiatric-faculty input, and that such input would also be available to 150 geriatric-medical faculties established nationally. We will assume that at least 100 of them will be located at institutions that will also have psychiatric training programs and that each of the 15 geropsychiatric training programs would also be located at such institutions. We believe that 2 faculty members would be the minimum number necessary to get any such program underway. This would mean that we would need a total of 200 academic geropsychiatric faculty. In addition, 1 geropsychiatric faculty member would be added to each of the remaining 200 psychiatric and 50 geriatric faculties. The total estimated need for academic geropsychiatrists would then be on the order of 450 positions. Based on previous experience, we anticipate that we would have to train 900 geropsychiatrists to allow for a 50-percent loss of trainees to community practice. (At this point we presuppose that there would be an active market for practicing geropsychiatrists.)

Thus training a complement of academic geropsychiatrists would produce, as a byproduct, 450 practicing geropsychiatrists. We would further assume that 25 percent of the academic geropsychiatrists' time would be spent in practice. This would provide a total practice complement of 562 FTEs of geropsychiatric practitioners (450 + 112).

The estimated need for geropsychiatrists in 1977 was 1,130. Were the group of academic geropsychiatrists trained, they would thus be able to meet about half of that need. If the remaining 50 percent were distributed between psychiatrists and geriatricians in a 2:1 ratio, it would require 380 FTEs of psychiatrists' time and 190 additional FTEs of geriatricians' time. This load might, in fact, be further dissipated by the potential use of other types of providers, such as psychologists, social workers, and nurse practitioners or physicians' assistants. This basic estimation technique can be applied to the future FTE needs projected here. The result is shown in table 6-1. This projection is clearly too static in the sense that the same number of academic geropsychiatrists are required each year, although the number of people trained by them grows sevenfold over the course of the time period described. Nonetheless, this kind of crude approximation gives us some sense that an additional 190 geriatricians might be needed today and that as many as 700 might be needed by the year 2030, simply to provide a portion of the geropsychiatric care.

Estimates Based on Prevalence of Mental Illness

At the same time, we appreciate that these data are based on an assumption that geropsychiatric care would be limited to only that care currently being provided by psychiatrists to persons over the age of 65. This may be a major

Table 6-1
Projection of Degree to Which Geropsychiatric Training Programs Will Meet the Need for Geropsychiatric Services

Type of Provider	Estimated Number of Providers Required			
	1977	1990	2010	2030
Academic geropsychiatrists	450 (112)[a]	450 (112)	450 (112)	450 (112)
Practicing geropsychiatrists	450	450	450	450
General psychiatrists	379	586	752	1400
Geriatricians	189	292	376	700
Total FTEs needed	1468	1778	2028	3000

[a] Twenty-five percent of faculty time estimated for patient care.

underestimation of the total amount of geropsychiatric care needed in the country both today and in the future. Thus we regard this analysis as a lower-bound estimate and now turn to a method of reaching an upper-bound estimate.

To achieve the latter, we approach the geropsychiatric personnel requirements by estimating the need for psychiatric care among the elderly. The prevalence of mental illness among persons aged 65 and older has been estimated to be 10 to 20 percent in various community surveys. (Carl Eisdorfer estimated 12 percent in a personal communication.) We can derive an estimate of the need for psychiatric services from (1) the prevalence of mental illness in the elderly (and we picked a low figure), (2) census figures, (3) a figure for the number of patient encounters per year per psychiatrist, and (4) the estimate by Birren and Sloane (1977) of six visits per patient per year. The latter requires examination.

The two most prevalent psychiatric conditions in the elderly are dementia and depression. The former requires an average of two visits for initial assessment and an average of two visits per year thereafter for crisis intervention. Depression requires at least three visits per year for drug management plus two per year for crisis intervention. A small number of patients with depression, paranoia, toxic psychoses, and other problems require a large number of visits for interactive ("talking") therapy; this would raise the average. Overall, this suggests an average number nearer five than six visits per year. The Psychiatry Practice Study Report (USC/DRME 1978) shows 40.1 encounters per week per psychiatrist. Assuming an average working year (subtracting vacations, illness, and time otherwise not practicing) of 47.4 weeks (Gaffney 1979), the psychiatrist has 1,901 encounters per year. The United States population aged 65 and older was 23,400,000 in 1977. If we take the lowest estimate of 10 percent with serious mental illness, and assume five visits per year for each patient, there are 11,700,000 visits needed. Dividing 11,700,000 by 1901, we calculate that 6,155 geropsychiatric FTEs are needed to provide the desired level of care.

Estimates Based on British Experience

We might be tempted to look for a manpower model in a society in which geriatrics and geriatric psychiatry are better developed. Typically, within the British National Health Service, six psychiatric-consultant posts are created per district of 200,000 population. Of these, an average of one will be a psychiatrist "with special interest in geriatrics." Thus, for the United States population in 1980, the requirement to match the British standard would be about 7,000 psychiatrists and about 1,200 geriatric psychiatrists. However, the allocation of all consultant posts in Britain is sparse compared with levels of specialist care in the United States. There are two important reasons for this difference: (1) the American people expect specialists to be widely available; (2) in the British system, access to a specialist exists only through a general practitioner.

We note that the United States has 25,000 psychiatrists rather than 7,000, as would be projected from the British figures. If the same 3.57:1 ratio were applied to the estimate of need for geriatric psychiatrists, then 4,300 of the latter would be needed to match the British level of services, corrected for cross-national difference.

Supply Considerations

Turning to supply, we find a marked shortfall against anticipated demand, or need. The AMA Physician Survey for December 31, 1977 indicates that 66 physicians nationwide listed both geriatrics and psychiatry among the three specialties they were allowed to mention. Because the response rate in this survey was 88 percent, this would project to possibly 75 self-identified geropsychiatrists in the United States. If we insist that geriatrics and psychiatry each be cited as either first or second in number of hours of self-identified activity per week, there were only 54 in the survey (or 61, corrected for the response rate). Persons listing geriatrics as one of their first three specialties who were also certified by the American Board of Psychiatry and Neurology numbered 17, or 26 percent. Of the psychiatrists, 45 percent were board certified (USC/DRME 1978). Among AMA respondents, 21 (or 32 percent) belonged to the American Psychiatric Association, compared with 60 percent of all psychiatrists. The fact that these percentages are "subnormal" among the self-identified geropsychiatrists suggests that a figure even lower than 61 or 75 should be taken as the figure for present-day, thoroughly competent, specialized geropsychiatrists. A panel of consultants has suggested from their own knowledge that the correct number is between 20 and 30 in the United States,[1] and the Birren-Sloane report (1977) estimates 20.

On the other hand, the situation may be changing. Carl Eisdorfer reports (personal communication) that 400 persons have joined the newly formed American Association for Geriatric Psychiatry; however, not all these members are from the medical profession. Nonetheless, we could find no evidence that this explosive "growth" is due to an increase in training programs. In fact, there is every evidence that this is not the case. Eisdorfer estimated (and our panel agreed) that the current capacity for output of geropsychiatric fellows is less than 20 per year. There are seven advanced geropsychiatric education programs in the country, according to our consultants (University of Washington, Duke, University of California at Los

Angeles, Rush–Presbyterian–St. Luke's [Chicago], Boston University, University of Pittsburgh, and University of Texas [Houston]). Only four of these actually give fellowship (that is, postresidency) training now; for the most part, this consists of six months during residency plus one year of fellowship. The faculty now in place have usually had just these eighteen months of specialized geropsychiatric training. One of the remaining universities offered fellowship training for the first time in July 1979. Another provides special training in geropsychiatry to psychiatry residents for three to six months of their entire residency. The seventh is still in the planning stage. As far as the panel was aware, these are the only sites in the country where specific training in geropsychiatry is available, even at the residency level.

Thus the need to mount educational programs is enormous. Recall that the current estimate of need, just for geropsychiatric faculty, is 700 persons and that the need ranges as high as 6,680, depending on how much of the direct-patient-care need is to be met by geropsychiatrists per se. By 2030 the latter figure would be closer to 15,000.

Eisdorfer felt that the goal should be to provide a sufficient number of geropsychiatrists to treat a large share of mental illness in the elderly. Yet this goal seems almost impossible to attain. He also recommended the rapid training of 50 new faculty members, after which about 50 additional fellows per year could be managed. Even if all positions were filled and there were no dropouts, this would produce only 65 geropsychiatrists per year. By 1990 there would be 650, ignoring the residual from the present handful. This number approaches the flow needed just to staff teaching hospitals. All consultants admitted that recruitment into geropsychiatry is difficult.

For these reasons, our panel, in contrast with Eisdorfer, argued that the mental-health needs of the elderly could not be met by means of fleshed-out geropsychiatry training and, furthermore, that this may not even be desirable. Almost all patients aged 65 and older with serious mental illness also have major physical impairments. Thus the well-trained geriatric specialist would be the ideal person to assume their care. It was argued that for only a small number of patients would the special expertise of a geropsychiatrist be needed, and that this could be obtained by consultation.

Thus the panel recommended that large numbers of geriatric specialists be recruited and trained. They felt that the challenge to provide modern mental-health care for the elderly could be met by such a specialist, but not by the internist or family physician with one to three months of geriatric training during his or her residency, and surely not by the general practitioner. They recommended that every teaching hospital with an internal-medicine, family-practice, or psychiatry residency, or more than one of these, should have geropsychiatric faculty and clinical teaching facilities; that each hospital with an internal-medicine or family-practice residency should develop a geriatric fellowship program; and that most of the geropsychiatric teaching effort should be directed toward the geriatric specialist and a minor amount toward the geropsychiatrist.

Each geropsychiatric program could train an average of one geropsychiatry fellow per year and could provide six months of geropsychiatry training for the geriatric-medicine fellows. Four geriatric specialists could thus receive their psychiatric component for every full-fledged geropsychiatrist produced. Each geriatric specialist could then be one-third the equivalent of a geropsychiatrist in terms of number of mental-health visits performed per year. Accordingly, this plan has 1.33 times the efficiency of training geropsychiatrists; more importantly, the product is more versatile and effective because of the mixture of abilities for dealing with mental and physical problems.

Note

1. The panel included Lissy Jarvik, M.D., Ph.D. (University of California at Los Angeles); Bruce Sloane, M.D. (University of Southern California); Manuel Straker, M.D. (Veterans Administration Hospital, Wadsworth).

7

The Evolution
of Geriatrics

So far we have addressed a series of projections about the anticipated need for geriatric services. In chapter 3, we argued that there exists a base of knowledge and skill sufficient to justify the identification of an area of concentrated effort. Whether geriatrics will or even should evolve as a distinct specialty is the focus of this chapter. Here we examine a variety of issues pertinent to discussions of how health care might be delivered to the elderly. A number of organizational and regulatory issues are raised including some of the barriers to active recruitment of needed health professionals into geriatrics. We offer a framework for assessing the desired rate of growth of the field, and we address directly the question of specialty status by drawing on the contrasting examples of two medical specialties: pediatrics and family practice. This question of specialty status is the source of considerable discussion. Even in England, where geriatrics has established a much stronger foothold, a debate is currently raging about whether geriatrics should continue as a distinct specialty or become more closely reidentified with general internal medicine (Stout 1979; Williamson 1979a, 1979b).

Geriatrics in Context

The manpower requirements described in the preceding chapters can be interpreted only as guideline estimates based on extrapolating various projections of utilization of services onto an assumedly constant means of supplying these services. Although we have examined the manpower implications of dividing the services to be delivered among several different kinds of providers in varying proportions, we have not looked intensively at ways in which the delivery system might be reorganized. A few remarks about the organization of geriatric services are in order at this point.

Several components of a desirable geriatric-care program are proposed. These building blocks, in turn, serve to foster a few cardinal principles that underlie the proposed system. A basic precept of the system is that the older person should remain autonomous to the greatest extent possible. This autonomy implies that community-based care will be a mainstay, with extensive efforts made to allow the elderly patient to live at home. (We must not lose sight of the important fact that most of the care of the elderly is provided not by professionals, but by family members and friends. This support system is the cornerstone for building supplemental professional services.)

Before we can establish an effective means of delivering community-based care programs in geriatrics, a number of additions and some changes must be made in our personnel. We currently lack the corps of providers needed to deliver care at home. This corps consists of both social- and medical-service providers, although the distinction may sometimes be arbitrary. It includes visiting nurses (of various levels), physiotherapists, occupational therapists (who work on activities of daily living), and social workers. From the medical perspective, the keystone of the delivery system may be a single, nonduplicated source of primary care.

Primary Care

American medicine continues to struggle with the question of how to make primary care available. In the model used here, we have distributed the primary care function among several different types of providers in varying proportions, but there is now no systematic means to ensure that (1) everyone has a source of primary care or (2) every person has only one source of such care. Because there is no system of capitation payment, those receiving no services (and some undefined portion of those receiving only specialized services) cannot be said to be getting primary care or to be accounted for in any list that might be compiled of those needing various types of services. At the same time, because specialists perceive themselves as offering primary-care services, other elderly persons may be receiving primary care from several different sources and might, therefore, appear on several lists of those in need.

If primary care is to be a central feature of American geriatric service, we have a variety of potential providers. Currently, such care is provided by a mixture of primary-care physicians and specialists (Aiken et al. 1979). In an unduplicated system of primary care, the organ-system subspecialist would be far less appropriate for the role. Using the British model of geriatric-medical services as a case in point, we have observed that one area of potential weakness in a system built around a primary-care source who calls in geriatric consultants as needed is the potential fracture of communications between the specialist and the general practitioner. The latter serves as the gatekeeper, and the former acts only upon his invitation. Under such an arrangement, the specialist may not be strongly motivated to try to improve the quality of primary care by direct feedback to the general practitioner. Problems due to missed diagnosis, overuse of medications, or similar errors of omission and commission will not be prevented in the absence of an active monitoring and communication system.

There seems no way in the near future that we could field a corps of geriatricians able to assume the full responsibility of primary care for the elderly, nor is it at all clear that such a path is desirable. The organ-system subspecialist lacks the interest and breadth to provide primary care for a particular age group; we are left, then, with the issue of whether such care can be provided adequately by existing types of primary-care providers or whether geriatrics requires special knowledge and skills at the primary-care level. Our review of the medical needs of the aged suggests that these needs are perhaps greatest at the primary-care level, where the recognition of problems in unusual presentations must be combined with the ability to mobilize a variety of community-based resources. Perhaps the ideal would be to identify a primary-care resource with special interest in the problems of the aged and ready access to a smaller (and therefore more feasibly developed) group of geriatric specialists.

One possible means of overcoming this difficulty in the United States would involve the extended use of providers that are more apparent in this country than in England, namely, new types of health professionals such as the geriatric nurse practitioner (GNP) and the physician's assistant (PA) (Scheffler et al. 1979). If much of the burden for the daily primary care of the elderly were undertaken by GNPs working under the supervision of geriatric specialists, an active linkage of primary and specialist geriatric care would be facilitated by direct-line responsibility.

Several modifications in current practice would be necessary before such a method of providing geriatric care would be possible. We lack sufficient GNPs and geriatric specialists. Current regulations would have to be amended to provide more direct-care authority (and commensurate reimbursement) for nurse practitioners and physician's assistants. Precedent for these changes is already set in the case of rural health care (Kane, Dean, and Solomon 1979).

Unfortunately, there has not been any surge of enthusiasm for geriatrics among nurses. Although the training and philosophy of nursing is eminently compatible with the spirit of geriatrics, nurses to date have been little more enthusiastic than physicians in flocking to the banner of geriatric care. Perhaps the expanded responsibilities offered by the proposed extensive role of the GNP in primary geriatric care may attract a cadre of nurses seeking to expand and thus enhance their careers. In England it has been possible (but not easy) to find a cadre of physicians who see geriatrics as a useful and rewarding career in medicine. The training posts in geriatrics, however, are not yet oversubscribed; the IOM report (1978) raises some questions about the quality of the physicians who seek geriatric posts in Britain. We anticipate that the same will hold true in this country, even if interest in geriatrics is stimulated by increased training opportunities and greater curriculum coverage in medical schools.

We have been quick to point out the need for both quantitative and qualitative improvements in care. The ready response to such deficiencies is a call for more and better programs of training. We would urge a similar cry for increased efforts in this area, but we also acknowledge that educational efforts alone will not be enough. Studies of the performance of health professionals suggest that they, like most groups, are sensitive to their environment (Kane, et al. 1976b; Hughes et al. 1974; Moscovice 1978). If we are to aim toward the improvement of geriatric care, it would be well to examine the incentives currently available to attract practitioners into the field and to offer the kind of care we feel is important.

Medical practice is generally paid for on the basis of units of service. There are essentially two models for this payment. Either payment is tied directly to units of service, as in fee-for-service medicine or cost reimbursement of hospitals and nursing homes, or a fixed amount is paid regardless of the specific amounts of individual care, as is the case with salaried practitioners or per-diem charges for institutions. Each of these approaches has its own strengths and weaknesses. Some critics have attacked the former as a perverse incentive system whereby the rewards are greater as the patient deteriorates and more resources must be expended. Conversely, the fixed-payment system has been portrayed as one in which the incentives are toward doing as little as possible in order to maximize profit. Given that the elderly may not exercise active consumer choice because they are either insecure about losing their present care resources (Olsen, Kane, and Kasteler 1976) or very dependent as institutional inmates, the economist's belief in the desirability of the free marketplace is hardly warranted. Regulation seems necessary to protect the consumer and the payor (often the government).

Unfortunately, regulation is unpopular and often ineffective. Because most of the approaches to regulation are based on concepts of structure and process, the thrust of these rules has generally been to ensure that some minimal set of services is provided. These demands for practice orthodoxy may be rightly interpreted as restrictive and often arbitrary.

A more satisfying approach would be less specific about the means of achieving a set of patient-care goals but would pay more attention to defining those goals precisely and to assessing whether or not they are achieved. We strongly endorse the concept of linking payments to outcomes, especially when those outcomes are tied to prognosis for individual patients or groups of patients. Such an approach would leave providers free to test a variety of therapeutic strategies and even to move outside traditional medical models to give more attention to the social aspects of geriatric care.

Clearly, the heart of such a system is the data that would offer a reasonably accurate forecast of the course of a geriatric patient. The development of this data base offers opportunities for important work in geriatrics. The existence of these opportunities and the lessons they offer for the practice of medicine in general (where the basic paradigms are the same) ought to provide incentives for professionals interested in working in this area.

It is easy to argue the importance of geriatrics and the contributions the field can make to meet the needs of an underserved group. In many ways, geriatrics epitomizes the World Health Organization conception of health. It addresses the social and mental areas of well-being as well as the physical. Data from geriatric-evaluation units provide two important lessons: (1) geriatric patients with multiple chronic problems are indeed capable of improving their level of functioning; (2) many of the problems these individuals face result either from overly enthusiastic treatment or from failure to identify important pathological processes.

If practitioners are to be attracted to geriatrics, a number of changes appear warranted. One important early step is to change the image of geriatric practice; long-term care is not a prestigious medical activity. Various remedies have been suggested. These include greater exposure of students and practitioners to the accomplishments possible in career geriatrics, the development of an active research agenda—including basic, clinical, and health services—evidence of interest in geriatrics by prestigious individuals, and the elevation of practice in this field to specialty status.

Unfortunately, although each of these activities is being pursued, none is underway at a level that would ensure success. However, one basis for optimism is the recent evidence of physician migration in response to market forces. Analyses of the geographic distribution of physicians have shown that many physicians, including a variety of specialists, have established practice in small rural towns (Schwartz et al. 1980). This migration appears to be, in large part, a response to the rapidly growing pool of physicians in urban areas and the subsequent saturation of opportunities for new practices in such areas.

Two lessons from this migration are especially germane for geriatric forecasting: (1) It is possible to saturate medical markets (despite the general shibboleth that, in medical care, supply creates demand); and (2) physicians are indeed responsive to these market forces, even to the point of geographic migration. It would thus seem feasible that some physicians in closely allied fields (medicine, psychiatry, family practice) might be susceptible to inducements to move laterally into geriatrics if those opportunities were properly presented and career pathways were established.

The experience in England adds further strength to this belief. The opportunities offered by careers in geriatrics were sufficiently enticing to a generation of specialist trainees to induce some of them to alter their goals. As consultant posts in geriatrics became available and similar positions in medicine did not, a cadre of well-trained geriatricians resulted. The situation in England has demonstrated that physicians can indeed find

the care of the elderly a professionally satisfying and intellectually challenging pursuit. Some caution is warranted, however. As the specialist/consul-
tant role as a whole has become less attractive in Britain, enrollment in
geriatric training has declined.

Nursing

In many respects, geriatric nursing has suffered from the same problems as
geriatric medicine: low prestige, poor pay, weak image. It is equally true
that nursing is responding along with medicine to the renaissance of interest
in the aged. One career area where these interests coincide is that of the
geriatric nurse practitioner (GNP). Historically the nursing profession has
been ambivalent about the practitioner movement and the extent to which it
is compatible with a larger nursing mission; nursing rejected the nurse-practitioner (NP) role when it was proffered by medicine on the grounds that
it represented an effort to ape the physician (Sadler, Sadler, and Bliss 1975).
Nursing has, in fact, taken up the term "gerontic nursing" to permit more
emphasis on the gerontologic components and to reinforce the distinction
from medical geriatrics (Gunter and Estes 1979).

The GNP represents an attractive means of providing primary-care services. The role promises a route to independent (but supervised) practice in
a mode that can emphasize the best of medicine and nursing as well as of
gerontology. There is, however, a series of significant, but not insurmount-
able, barriers to effective use of geriatric nurse practitioners. A major problem is payment. Although several states provide for Medicaid payment for
services rendered by midlevel practitioners (physician's assistants [PAs] and
NPs), Medicare will pay only for those services performed under on-site
supervision of a physician. This policy severely threatens extensive use of
the GNP, especially because Medicare Part B payments cover the bulk of
costs for physician services for much of the elderly population, including
those covered by Medicaid. A precedent has been established for the direct-
cost reimbursement of NP or PA services (if supervised by a physician who
makes at least periodic on-site visits) under the Rural Health Services Clinic
Act (PL 95-210) on the grounds that rural people lack adequate access to
primary care. A similar argument might be readily made for the elderly, and
adequate safeguards could be developed to prevent abuse.[1]

The second area of difficulty is the need to amend licensure laws and
regulations to allow NPs to practice, including prescribing from a limited
formulary. Activity on this front varies from state to state, but sufficient
models exist to offer means to overcome this problem if there is a supportive political environment. (Because PAs operate under a Medical Practice

Act rather than a Nurse Practice Act, they may be less restricted in this regard in many states).

If these barriers are removed, it seems reasonable to anticipate marked growth in the development of GNP programs. Although it may be overoptimistic to expect a stampede of applicants, there is reasonable cause for predicting that the GNP role will appeal to a substantial number of nurses who see it as an opportunity to fulfill a variety of career and personal goals.

Long-Range Plans for Training Geriatricians

We have noted the benefits that medical personnel with good geriatric training could provide in geriatric research, medical teaching, and service delivery to the elderly. Currently few people are specifically trained for any of these career specialties, and training resources in both money and expertise are quite limited. Even our most modest goals require many more geriatric specialists. Decisions must be made along two dimensions. First, how quickly should we try to close the gaps? Second, should training proceed in stages or in steady proportions? In the staged approach, only academics are initially trained; these trainees then train practitioners. By contrast, the steady-proportions approach constantly trains about the same fraction of academicians and practitioners.

It may seem natural to combat poor care for the elderly by investing in a crash program to train academicians, but this approach presents obstacles. Every component of the production process imposes limits on the size of high-quality programs and on the speed at which they can be implemented.

The initial cadre of teachers will generally not have received much specialized geriatric training; in the early years of the program, they will be learning along with the fellows. As the goal for the number of initial faculty grows, the additional members found may be less and less well qualified for the task. The training programs can be expected to improve as time goes by, so that the earliest fellows may not get training as good as that provided to later fellows. Moreover, we can expect the pace of geriatric research to pick up as researchers are trained and new institutions tried. Early concepts may quickly become obsolete. These are all arguments for a gradual buildup of programs.

The medical students graduating in any given year vary in their talents and interests. Because we want to encourage all kinds of interest in geriatric medicine, it would be indefensible to try to channel all geriatric recruits in the 1980s into academic work and those in the 1990s into practice. If academic programs select for talent, they will necessarily have fewer fellows than applicants. Without extensive raiding of other fields, finding a very large group of high-quality applicants will be difficult. Another problem with a staged approach is that the medical-school cohort of academicians will be a large group, all the same age. This will prevent a proper blending of junior and senior workers and will be discouraging to future people trying to enter geriatric medicine, who will have to wait many years for tenured slots to open.

Institutional reasons against the staged approach and against creating huge temporary programs can also be cited. A steady program with constant goals is easier to manage, and the people in it can develop skills with the confidence that they can continue to use them. Recruitment of high-quality faculty is easier if programs are expected to last more than a few years. There is a standard, well-understood way of training fellows and residents; the radical changes in this method that would be necessary to train large numbers of people quickly in only a few settings my not work. Finally, because turning the crash programs off may be difficult, there may be a glut of academic geriatric specialists in a few decades.

Although the first few academic geriatric trainees will be extremely useful, so will the first few practicing geriatricians. Because service delivery is particularly important in geriatrics, feedback from those in practice about the value of training and new ideas developed in practice will add to their worth as better-trained practitioners. Historically, half or more of the fellows trained for academic medicine end up in community practice, so the academic approach automatically satisfies some of this need. We must ask, however, whether the training that the 50 percent who do not stay in academia receive is best suited to their future work. More realism in program goals, and perhaps earlier identification of what the fellows will ultimately do, may result in training that is better tailored to their individual needs.

Leaving aside these practical considerations, other theoretical arguments can be marshaled against a completely staged buildup. The economically analogous choice is between investment and consumption, where academicians are considered an investment and practitioners a consumption benefit for the elderly. A standard economic example is corn. Suppose we have developed a more nutritious variety of corn, but have only a little of it. We must decide whether to put it all into seed or whether we can give some of it out now and put the rest into seed. The problem is usually handled by considering the set of all feasible consumption streams and picking the one that has maximum utility value. Under many assumptions, the best path has more investment in the early stages, but has at least some consumption throughout. The exact answer depends on several factors. More early consumption is desirable when there is no good substitute for the first few units of new corn, when the threshold of satiation for new corn is low, when the productivity of seed is low, or when society places greater value on current consumption than on future consumption. The medical analogs are (1) whether the first few community practitioners can meet the bulk of specialized needs so that additional practitioners will handle primarily the same problems that less-specialized physicians could care for; (2) how productive teachers are in training more practitioners; and (3) how society values the health of today's elderly as opposed to the health of those in 2010.

The economic argument against crash programs is simply the wastefulness of straining resources beyond their natural limit. To get the last units of output, either quality has to fall or many more resources have to be expended. The problems of the elderly are pressing, but not so pressing that we would want to take large amounts of ill-suited resources from other fields of medicine in order to save a little time in achieving our goals.

Pediatrics and Family Practice: Lessons for Geriatric Medicine

In developing a strategy for implementing new educational programs in geriatric medicine and analyzing the importance of formal specialty recognition, a useful perspective can be obtained by examining analogs from other specialties. We will therefore examine the forces that led to the development of pediatrics and family practice in this nation. In contrast to many specialties developed on the basis of new technology, these two were organized around service functions, one of them being age related.

Stevens (1971) identified two cogent arguments in favor of specialization. By allowing some specialization of activity, a specialty is able to contribute additional knowledge in a field. Concentration of interest in a particular area often leads to improved services in that field. She goes on to describe the steps that specialties follow during the process of their evolution and that eventually lead to their inclusion in the medical curriculum. These steps include specially identified faculty, distinctive residency and fellowship programs, and some form of speciality recognition.

The first step involves an informal socialization of individuals interested in a common field and sharing scientific and intellectual activities. This banding together is followed by the development of formal organizations, the appearance of practitioners limiting their practice to that field, and emerging concerns about the standards of knowledge in the field. Next may come the establishment of limited numbers of faculty positions, including special chairs, and demands for inclusion of field elements in the continuum of medical education. Special programs, an accreditation process, and specialty certification eventually occur.

Pediatrics

Pediatrics began to evolve in the 1850s, partly because of an awakened interest in the welfare of children and their special needs. The first White House Conference on Children was held in 1909 and was followed by the founding of the Children's Bureau in 1912. The major advances in public health and biochemistry in the late 1800s and early 1900s generated increased scientific interest in the care of children. The first full-time chairmanship of a pediatric department was established at the Johns Hopkins University 1912 and became an important force in the development of research in the field.

The American Pediatrics Society, primarily an academic organization, was formed in 1887, shortly after the identification of a special AMA section on pediatrics. It is perhaps pertinent to note that an editorial in the *Journal of the American Medical Association* in 1896 stated that pediatrics should never become a specialty because it was really part of the whole of medicine.

Federally supported maternal- and infant-care programs began in the early 1920s, and by 1930 there were reported to be approximately 1,500 full-time and 2,000 part-time pediatricians. The American Academy of Pediatrics, founded in 1930 as an action group, became a potent force for the inclusion of pediatrics in the medical curriculum, the identification of separate pediatric beds in hospitals, the establishment of special outpatient clinics, and the need for specialty certification in pediatrics. The American Board of Pediatrics was founded in 1933, facilitating the accreditation of standardized residency programs and specialty certification for the individual physician.

Family Practice

The evolutionary process of pediatrics was slow and methodical in contrast to that of family practice almost half a century later. The evaluation of family practice as a specialty followed a very different pathway (Chisholm 1978; Pisacano 1978). For most of the history of medical practice, general practice (the forerunner of family practice) was the predominant mode; but the situation began to shift in the second quarter of the twentieth century. Between 1931 and 1963 the number of general practitioners declined from

90 per 100,000 population to 37 per 100,000; by 1971, the ratio had fallen to 24 general practitioners per 100,000 population. In 1931, 83 percent of American physicians were general practitioners, most without formal post-graduate preparation beyond the internship. But the balance was shifting; by 1940, 24 percent were specialists (Severinghaus 1965).

These events, together with the general practitioners' "lack of prestige" in academic medical centers and their increasing difficulties in obtaining hospital privileges, were factors in the founding of the American Academy of General Practice (AAGP) in 1947.[2] This body was developed by practitioners to promote recognition of the quality of general practice and to preserve the practice privileges of its members. One means of accomplishing this end was to work toward specialty status for the general practitioner.

Working within the context of organized medicine, the academy's leaders began a steady campaign toward this goal. The American Medical Association supported strengthening the postgraduate training of general practitioners. In 1950 the AMA approved the first residency training programs in general practice, but many of these positions went unfilled. In 1959, a group supported by neither the AAGP nor the AMA chartered the American Board of General Practice; without such backing, however, nothing came of the effort. At the same time, public and professional sentiment was growing to favor strongly some type of effort to increase the availability of primary care (U.S. DHEW 1959; Darley 1961; WHO 1963). A series of national commissions (Millis 1966; Willard 1966; National Commission on Community Health Service 1966) echoed the need for a renaissance of primary care and identified the family practitioner as a means of achieving such care.

The AAGP worked closely with the AMA to develop joint recommendations for the establishment of a distinct specialty of family practice. In 1967, the draft proposal by the AAGP for board certification received encouragement from the Advisory Board of Medical Specialties (now the American Board of Medical Specialties). The following year the essentials for residency training programs in family medicine were drafted by an ad hoc committee composed of representatives of the AAGP, the AMA's Council on Medical Education, and its Section Council for General Practice.

In 1969 the American Board of Family Practice was approved by the American Board of Medical Specialties upon recommendation of the Liaison Committee for Special Boards. The initial roster of the fifteen-member American Board of Family Practice was broadly representative of practicing general practitioners from across the country. Few represented an academic constituency of family practice, although most of the five members representing the other major specialties (internal medicine, pediatrics, surgery, obstetrics and gynecology, psychiatry and neurology) had strong

associations with academic medicine. The Society of Teachers of Family
Medicine was formed in 1967 but did not begin its rapid growth until after
the founding of the specialty and the subsequent investment of substantial
federal resources to support the development of family-practice programs
in medical schools at both the undergraduate and postgraduate levels.

The resultant growth has been dramatic. The family-practice training
programs originally approved have now expanded to more than 350
residency programs. Departments of family practice exist in most medical
schools; only a few have no academic unit at all. This rapid growth pro-
voked a series of problems for the academic community. Faculty were con-
scripted from two major sources: (1) academicians in other fields of
primary (and occasionally specialty) care, and (2) community practitioners
of family or general practice. In both instances, the transition was difficult;
only recently has family practice begun to consolidate the necessary
academic base with an effort toward establishing an appropriate balance
among teaching, service, and research. For many in the academic
community, the failure of family practice to undertake research has jeopar-
dized its position as an academic discipline.

Geriatrics

Taken together, pediatrics and family practice represent examples of the
two primary pathways toward the creation of a new specialty. Pediatrics
evolved from an academic base, gaining support from practicing specialists
as they became available. Family practice was the product of a practicing
constituency who saw specialty status as a means of averting their extinc-
tion; the academic component grew only after the political battles were
won.

The historical evolution of geriatrics has taken a different course thus
far from either of these two primary-care specialties. Considerable interest
of a cyclic nature in geriatric medicine has been evident for many decades.
In the late 1800s and early 1900s, the first stirrings were identifiable in
North America. The first American textbook of geriatric medicine was
published in 1914 by L.L. Nascher, who was also credited with having
invented the word *geriatrics*. The interest waned and disappeared during
World War I and resurfaced only for a relatively brief period in the late
1920s and early 1930s. It has been suggested that physicians were reluctant
to enter geriatrics because of its lesser interest as compared with other fields
and because of economic difficulty in developing viable practices. The
elderly were correctly perceived as having less money and more illness than
the remaining population.

In the early 1940s, a new upsurge of public interest in the status of the elderly and the diseases of old age was noted. This renaissance led to the formation of two societies concerned with the elderly population: the American Geriatric Society in 1942 and the Gerontological Society in 1945. The former was composed of physicians, whereas the latter served a broader constituency. The founding of these two societies was coincident with the recognition that almost 7 percent of the population was over age 65. During this time there was a realization that the care of the elderly was a multidisciplinary process involving educational, medical, sociological, economic, and religious fields.

Once more the flurry of activity was short lived, and only in the 1960s was there a reawakening of concern for the elderly. This concern finally led to the passage in 1965 of the amendment to the Social Security Act known as Medicare. Curiously, even this massive infusion of funds into the medical care of the elderly did not stimulate an academic response. As late as 1977, the American Geriatric Society opposed a separate specialty (Reichel 1977). Only very recently has a special nucleus of physicians interested in the elderly emerged and a locus developed in the health-professional schools for a gerontological and geriatric component within the curriculum (see chapter 2). The history of geriatric medicine has been one of constant reinvention.

Several hypotheses explain why geriatric medicine has until now failed to carve out a niche for itself in the health professions. The first is organizational. Although formal geriatric and gerontological societies were founded more than thirty years ago, their character and composition have been different from those of comparable organizations in other specialties. These geriatric societies have been multidisciplinary, and multidisciplinary societies have usually been less effective in accomplishing their goals than unidisciplinary societies. Within them, geriatric medicine has not had representation from academic medicine's power structure.

A second hypothesis is that research on clinical issues in geriatrics has been slow to develop, although gerontology as a basic science has been quite active for two decades. The analogy to pediatrics surfaces again; research on the characteristic health problems of children (such as infectious diseases or dehydration in infants) was an important force in the evolution of pediatrics and its acceptance as an academic and practice specialty.

A third hypothesis is simply that ageism is a barrier to attracting enough physicians who wish to be identified as geriatricians. If one does not especially enjoy working with the elderly, one is more likely to remain a family physician, a general internist, or a psychiatrist rather than to take up geriatrics or geropsychiatry. This often seems to be true today, even when geriatric patients predominate in a physician's practice. We interviewed several internists, general practitioners, and family physicians whose practices were almost totally geriatric but who neither identified themselves as geriatricians in the AMA Physicians Survey nor became members of the American Geriatrics Society.

What evidence of the emergence of a geriatric specialty can be discerned in 1979?

1. A small group of physicians who identify themselves as geriatric specialists and geriatric faculty is emerging.
2. An increasing number of educational programs in geriatric medicine exist (at varying stages of development). There are two endowed chairs in geriatric medicine (at Cornell and at the Medical University of South Carolina).
3. Increasing amounts of funding are available for biomedical research on the special problems of the elderly (but insufficient funding exists for health-services research relevant to the elderly population).
4. Discussions are underway concerning the development of stronger professional associations in geriatric medicine and nursing—perhaps comparable to the associations of university professors in other specialties. Based on the earlier discussion, it is important to develop these stronger professional groupings with major involvement of the academic community.
5. Some financial support has been provided for developing a cadre of physicians and other health professionals with special knowledge of the problems of the elderly. However, the support is inadequate and threatens to create a situation in which the service needs may dominate the training effort.

This brief historical review offers a few important lessons. The data presented in chapter 2 suggest that there is a much smaller practicing constituency available for geriatrics than was the case for general or family practice. Moreover, there is not, at present, the groundswell of support for distinct specialty recognition among the formal organizations representing geriatrics. For example, the American Geriatrics Society reflects the IOM's approach of emphasizing a geriatrics education rather than developing a separate specialty (Reichel 1977). It is thus more likely that support for specialty status will come from the academic ranks as geriatric faculty are trained and recruited. In this regard, the evolution of a specialty in geriatrics, if it occurs, is more likely to resemble the path of pediatrics than that of family practice.

Regardless of the specialty designation, however, training programs in geriatrics will require faculty and they, in turn, will require preparation distinct from that primarily oriented toward clinical care. A lesson may be learned from the evolution of family practice as a specialty in recent times.

If geriatric medicine is to take its place at the academic table, then a cadre of individuals who are both clinically competent and capable of creative research is surely needed. The present dearth of faculty to lead emerging geriatric units is a major manifestation of this deficiency.

If geriatrics is to succeed academically, it must learn the lessons of family practice and establish active research programs that can form the basis of fellowship training. Such research will offer the means for faculty retention and promotion within the university; stressing the intellectual base of geriatric medicine will contribute proof that it is an interesing special area and will enhance its image as a discipline. This, in turn, will positively affect the attitudes and effectiveness of future generations of physicians.

Notes

1. Before we rush to implement a geriatric program based on the Rural Health Services Clinic Act, we would be wise to review the experiences of rural clinics. The administrative and regulatory load imposed by this law has been enormous. Fears of exploitation have produced very restrictive regulations that inhibit the spirit, if not the letter, of the law.

2. This group was renamed the American Academy of Family Physicians in 1972.

8 Development of a Curriculum in Geriatrics

This chapter addresses the prerequisites for the development of institutional programs for education, research, and service in geriatrics, together with the issue of how the desired types of personnel should be educated. Alternative modes of staffing the necessary educational programs are discussed, as well as problems anticipated in the implementation.

Strategy

Lessons can be drawn from the history of curriculum development and from observations on how geriatrics is taught in England, where it is more established. One obvious point is too often neglected. At a time when medical-school curricula are overcrowded, any new material must be inserted at the cost of something removed. With curriculum time at a premium, new programs, even in areas of identified need, may not be welcomed by the faculty. Success is unlikely without the support of key individuals in both the administrative and intellectual hierarchies. A new geriatric program must have strong support by the dean's office of the health-professional schools, particularly the schools of medicine and nursing, and by the senior administrative figures at other institutions such as long-term-care facilities and community-service centers that form part of the total program. If Rogers' (1980) predictions for the 1980s are close to the mark, it will be a time of little growth in academic medicine. New programs will have to displace existing ones. Programs offering personal care may have great difficulty competing with those using income-generating technology. Thus geriatrics will need active support if it is to germinate in this farmed-out soil.

Similarly, success is more likely when an institution can demonstrate commitment by the key leadership in internal medicine, family practice, psychiatry, and neurology, and in comparable divisions within the nursing faculty such as the nurse-practitioner programs. These commitments must involve a willingness to define the overall goals of a geriatric program and the specific behavioral objectives of its educational content.

In our view, faculty commitment must include a willingness to offer geriatric instructional material in all phases of the educational continuum, including several offerings in the undergraduate curriculum at both the pre-clinical and clinical levels; geriatric training for house staff in internal medicine, family practice, and psychiatry; and special fellowships in geriatrics-gerontology with an aim toward developing both competent faculty and clinicians wishing to specialize in this field. Finally, continuing medical-education programs should be offered.

In schools of nursing, we would envisage the introduction of geriatric content into the undergraduate curriculum, the development of geriatric-nurse-practitioner programs, and efforts to develop advanced programs in gerontological nursing as a future source of faculty leadership in this field.

Our own experience with the introduction of new clinical components into the curriculum strongly argues that effective adoption at the under-graduate level requires the presence of an established graduate program. The house staff serve as important role models for the undergraduate medical students, and their presence in the field provides important reinforcement even to the preclinical students. Equally important, the existence of a strong house staff program enhances the credibility of a new program in the eyes of faculty. Some new programs introduced into the curriculum have faded into oblivion for lack of adequate faculty support and appropriate practice opportunities after the course offering was completed. (The recent disbanding of departments of community medicine illustrates this phenomenon.) Because geriatrics is so pervasive in the practice of medicine, students must identify a full track that they can pursue throughout their under-graduate and graduate medical education.

An alternative is to follow the British example and focus most of the effort at the undergraduate level. Although anecdotal evidence suggests that graduates of the English medical schools have an improved understanding of the problems of the elderly, few of them have entered advanced training programs leading to the production of faculty for the academic departments of geriatrics and of consultants in geriatrics for the National Health Service. In England, advanced geriatric training programs have been unable to fill their positions with English-trained physicians and thus have had to rely on a large non-English-born component of trainees.

Other reasons can be advanced for concentrating efforts at the graduate level. Graduate students are more likely to stay in geriatrics and, it is hoped, in academic geriatrics, the area of greatest immediate need. Academic geriatricians are essential if geriatric medicine is to achieve rapid recognition as a legitimate academic discipline providing faculty for medical schools and teaching hospitals.

On the other hand, focusing efforts at the graduate level has some real dangers. We have already alluded to the pressures on the undergraduate curriculum. Undue emphasis on graduate training can distract attention and relieve the pressures for inclusion of geriatrics–gerontology in the under-graduate curriculum. Especially in a field such as geriatrics where much of the teaching takes place outside the traditional university hospital, a real and present danger is that the teaching program will remain outside the mainstream of medical education or will be given a small seat on the bench at the far end of the table.

To a large extent this has been the fate of many geriatric training programs in England. They tend to be housed in peripheral buildings away from the major teaching centers. (This exile phenomenon is often compounded by housing these programs in former workhouses, which reinforces the image of second-class status for geriatrics.) When the undergraduate teaching hours are shared with other services, the logistical problems of getting from morning to afternoon bases further frustrate the student. If geriatrics is to be an effective influence on student attitudes, the parent institution must give a clear message that geriatrics is valued enough to keep it within the mainstream.

For these reasons, we would elect to develop initial strength in the postgraduate years and, at the same time, work with the faculty in both the preclinical and clinical years to increase emphasis on geriatric-related material and sensitivity to the issues faced in providing care to the elderly. The residents and advanced trainees (fellows and junior faculty) would serve as teachers and role models for subsequent cohorts of medical students.

Because we believe that a significant part of the training for geriatric medicine will involve team interaction, we find the graduate-training strategy more effective. Graduate students can spend extended periods of uninterrupted time in the training program, rather than moving in and out to fit their schedules in other classes. Sustained time commitments of this nature are required for the development of team skills. These arguments would hold in selecting graduate-student-level trainees over undergraduate trainees in the other health-professional disciplines such as nursing, dentistry, social welfare, and occupational or physical therapy.

Where to Begin

To begin at the beginning, let us outline several steps in the development of a geriatric curriculum. Although the process is essentially similar to that for any new teaching enterprise, there are a few geriatric wrinkles.

An important first step is to define the roles and needs for the various types of health professionals required to implement a better system of care for the elderly on a state, regional, or national basis. This effort will serve as a basis for ongoing curricular planning, curricular adjustments, and implementation of programs.

With these estimates in hand, one can describe various health-professional roles important to the development of better health care for the elderly. For example, included within the physician stream are academic geriatricians required to fill the many faculty positions springing up in the field and to serve as potential leaders in geriatric medicine who would assume responsibility for the operation of large institutions important to the field. Among these institutions are intermediate- and long-term-care units in VA medical centers and large public or private long-term-care facilities.

These practice models of geriatric health professionals aid in the development of educational objectives expressed in terms of expected behaviors to be demonstrated by students. Our own experience would suggest that such behavioral objectives can be most readily developed for the most advanced health professionals (for example, in geriatric fellowship programs) and subsequently modified to address the introduction of geriatric medicine into the generalist stream of graduate training programs in internal medicine, family practice, and psychiatry. They can also serve as a framework for introducing new curricular materials and experiences into the undergraduate curriculum and as a conceptual focus for developing educational materials for other health-professional students. These efforts deserve a multispecialty and interdisciplinary effort, including the valuable contributions of social scientists with expertise in gerontology.

Once consensus on behavioral objectives is reached, the resources required to implement the various levels of educational and training curricula can be identified. These resources are to some extent traditional, but more frequently nontraditional for the usual academic medical center because they involve nursing homes, residential communities for the elderly, community-sited health and welfare centers, home-care organizations, and day hospitals.

One force in shaping the curriculum is the availability of faculty resources. Therefore, design of the curriculum should involve a prior inventory of both institutionally and community-based persons engaged in gerontological and geriatric research and service.

Development of curricular plans for educational programs, particularly at the undergraduate level, must involve faculty participation through mechanisms such as deans' committees. These lend overall support and credibility during the acceptance and implementation process. Plans for evaluation of the effectiveness of curricular innovations must be developed, with initial emphasis on the evaluation of those trainees who are deemed most important in a given institution's program.

Content of a Geriatric Curriculum

Proposing a specific set of items for inclusion in the content of any geriatric curriculum is beyond the scope of this book. Moreover, it is unrealistic to expect that any single set of such items would be universally accepted. The IOM has referred to material that is worthy of serious consideration, and several training programs have already begun to formulate educational objectives for geriatric graduates at various stages of training.

Here we introduce a few concepts that may prove helpful in the process of developing a curriculum in geriatrics. In the main these concepts are not unique to geriatrics. In appendixes C and D, we offer some examples of educational objectives designed for different levels of students in geriatrics. These are intended solely as examples to illustrate the conceptual points raised here.

Defining what should be learned and deciding how to teach it are two distinct processes. It is very valuable to articulate the former, thus allowing greater flexibility in the latter. We strongly endorse the concept of educational objectives expressed as behaviors to be demonstrated in the program graduates (Mager 1962).

A useful sequence is to think first of the behaviors sought in the most advanced graduate. These objectives will be the most complete and can be used as a source for more modest objectives for individuals who will receive substantially less training. This approach creates a cascading phenomenon in which the objectives for the most junior trainee are subsumed into those for more senior trainees. An example of this process is shown in appendix D, where a subset of the objectives designed for geriatric fellows can be used as a basis for objectives for medical residents, who might have a limited clinical and academic exposure to geriatrics as part of their overall training program. These in turn could be further modified into objectives for medical students.

With such objectives in hand, geriatric-program advocates will be better able to assess the current state of the undergraduate curriculum and to identify elements that are inadequately covered. A catalog of these acknowledged deficiencies provides a strong rationale for faster curricular reform.

A similar approach can be readily used in developing objectives for other health personnel. There are likely to be large areas of overlap. One recurrent item in most lists of objectives is the need for skills in team care. Team training poses a number of logistical problems despite its intuitive attraction. Levels of relative training must be well balanced; schedules must be coordinated and appropriate clinical experiences identified. It is not at all clear that team training, as contrasted with training for teamwork, is a desirable goal in undergraduate education. It may be more useful to concentrate efforts at this time on developing professionally appropriate skills that will allow the professional to contribute to a team effort in the future. At the same time, the rationale for teamwork in geriatric care should be emphasized as a curricular topic.

Problems in Implementing Geriatric Programs

A group committed to the introduction of geriatric curricular material must wrestle with the issue of whether geriatric–gerontology encompasses a special area of knowledge, skills, and attitudes and must be prepared to convince other faculty of this. Earlier portions of this book attest to our conviction that an increasingly substantial knowledge base has developed over the last decade in molecular biology, biochemistry, pharmacology, and other basic sciences, as well as in the behavioral and social sciences. Thus the medical care of the elderly can be approached on the same scientific basis as any other special area. In addition, the clinical skills required to manage the geriatric patient are distinctive, particularly those needed to mobilize and manage the various resources in the community. When questions of content are raised, it may be necessary to respond in clear detail with an enumeration of the knowledge, attitudes, and skills that constitute geriatric practice. In this connection, having defined behavioral objectives can lend clarity and force to this effort.

At present and for the foreseeable future, new geriatric programs will encounter a dearth of qualified faculty. As with many new enterprises, the founding faculty will have to be begged, borrowed, and stolen from other pursuits. This shortage, although serious in its own right, is disastrous if there is a lack of depth. Faculty inexperienced in geriatrics, academic medicine, or both are far less productive and far more insecure. There is a keen need, then, to think in terms of a critical mass of faculty sufficient to launch and sustain a teaching program. Previous experience suggests that the critical minimum for a medical school is probably three physicians supported by others with related skills, but there is little empirical data available to substantiate this assertion.

The pool of potential faculty is not large at the moment. Even if we are prepared to go to the practicing geriatrician as a source of faculty, the supplies are extremely limited. The AMA Physician Survey referred to elsewhere in this book reveals that only a small number of self-identified geriatricians perceive caring for the elderly as their primary mission. Similarly, the best estimates can identify only twenty to thirty physicians in the nation with formal training in geropsychiatry.

One of the first problems that program developers will have to confront in dealing with both colleagues and students is likely to be a set of attitudes about the elderly and those treating them. Butler (1975) has labeled this prejudice "ageism." Until recently, the aged have been a rather hidden part of our society. Caring for this population has been a relegated task rather than a sought-after one. The image of the geriatrician thus has not been a very positive one. Because the problems of the aged are so multifaceted and their etiology so multifactorial, traditional medical approaches have not been directly appropriate. The care of the elderly has, to a large extent, been seen as something left to physicians who have grown old with their patients or to a small group of practitioners who seek to profit from public funds such as Medicare and Medicaid. There is, in fact, an ironic paradox here. One hears academicians discuss geriatrics as a subject more appropriate for people other than physicians and then, almost simultaneously, argue that geriatrics is already being adequately and appropriately taught, and that much of what is now carried under that label is, in fact, the kind of thing that any well-trained internist, family physician, or psychiatrist already does.

This paradox reflects in part a very real concern about issues of territoriality. Internal medicine has recently been challenged by family practice in a battle over claims to the territory of primary care. Geriatrics could be viewed as another venture into the nonpediatric primary-care territory. There is genuine and well-founded concern about the possible infringement of a new cadre of geriatricians on established educational and practice patterns. The established specialties are apprehensive about geriatric medicine's role and the danger that it might reduce their clinical-practice base. Particularly in light of demographic predictions that a large percentage of the adult population will fall into what may be labeled the geriatric age range, the identification of a new group of specialists can be threatening indeed.

There are further similarities to the medical schools' recent dalliance with primary care. As with family practice, geriatrics implies the development of settings in environments and institutions that are not usually associated with academic medicine. In the case of geriatrics, these may be institutions that have not previously had any active association with health-professional schools. Examples of these types of institutions would include long-term-care facilities (especially nursing homes), multipurpose senior centers designed to provide social services in the community, day centers and other types of centers for the well elderly, community screening and counseling centers for the frail but coping elderly, old-age homes, and home-care programs. Nor is it realistic to expect that these facilities will all leap eagerly to forge new alliances with the academic centers. For the service-oriented institutions, these new relationships raise important issues about additional costs that the facilities must bear as a result of taking on a teaching role. Equally important, they raise more subtle, but very real, fears about loss of institutional autonomy and the possible impact that research may have on established patterns of activity.

Although there is currently an eruption of federal and private support to assist in the founding of major university-based efforts in geriatrics, the long-term survival of these programs will depend heavily on the development of adequate resources—both financial and structural. The familiar, but unresolved, task of balancing educational and service efforts must be struggled with and redefined anew with regard to the elderly population. New expectations will be raised, and the number of new types of providers recruited will not fit comfortably into the traditional faculty-advancement scheme. Once again, several lessons can be drawn from the experience with primary care.

There is a need to provide for more effective modes of delivering service and establishing models for teaching service delivery. This will entail new configurations of both inpatient and outpatient facilities. One can identify units such as the geriatric-evaluation unit (GEU) as an important adjunct to the more traditional hospital teaching service. New forms of ambulatory care will include ways of merging social and medical services at the primary-care level and the establishment of new types of ambulatory settings such as the day hospital. It will be more feasible in most instances to establish these innovative programs in settings other than the traditional teaching hospitals. The neophyte geriatric unit must then struggle with the question of how to establish innovative models on the one hand, and, on the other, remain visible in the mainstream of academic institutional life. The latter is not simply a selfish desire to be a part of a prestigious setting but is also a necessity if the program is to reach the undergraduate and graduate health professionals on more than a short-term basis.

This dilemma of being within and without has not been resolved by family practice and will be an important issue for geriatrics. The latter may have some advantage in that more of its efforts can and should be directed toward developing more effective means of delivering *inpatient* care. Because units such as the GEUs offer promise of improving the efficiency of the hospital's functioning, they may be intrinsically attractive to the institution and thus provide an active base of practice for geriatrics within the more traditional academic setting. This opportunity could provide an effective linkage into the more innovative ambulatory settings in peripheral locations.

Newly developing programs in geriatrics will encounter a lack of curricular materials. Historically, almost all new frontiers in medical education have been faced with the same problem of less than ideal educational materials to use as a base for developing their training programs. It is reasonable to expect that both the quality and quantity of these materials will increase as the market for them grows and the number of academicians working in the area expands. Nonetheless, the short-term scarcity of high-quality curricular materials threatens to limit the rapid development of educational programs. A response to this dilemma would be the active sharing of materials as they are developed and tested through some form of clearinghouse mechanism. The VA has recently concluded a contract for this purpose (Robbins et al. 1981). Several other projects through the Administration on Aging and the National Institute on Aging will support work related to this goal.

Geriatric academic efforts will be inhibited by lack of adequate financial support for both faculty and trainees. In our present period of no-growth budgets, new sources of support for faculty specifically dedicated to geriatric medicine are needed. A geriatric program lacking this institutional support may find itself attempting to support such activities through intensive clinical programs. Although the clinical base is a prerequisite for any successful program in geriatrics, an early overcommitment into this area may produce an imbalance that will drain faculty and trainee resources at precisely the time when they should be directed toward establishing the foundations of a sound academic program. We have already noted that current support for numbers of trainees would not be sufficient to meet the projected faculty needs.

In addition to the impetus of a strong faculty, introduction of geriatrics into the curriculum will require the support of the student body. The current level of student enthusiasm for primary care and humanistically oriented subjects may produce a mood of greater receptivity to geriatrics among the students. There is some evidence to suggest that students are becoming increasingly aware of the demographic transition in this country. To the extent that geriatric material can be offered as being broadly related to the practice of medicine in general, rather than as an inducement to enter geriatrics as a specialty, it is likely to be more enthusiastically supported by the student group. In essence, a soft-sell rather than a hard-sell approach is likely to be more effective.

An inevitable problem in establishing a new area of academic medicine will be the recruitment of adequate numbers of high-caliber advanced trainees. The experiences of programs in England suggest substantial difficulties in recruiting trainees other than foreign medical graduates into geriatrics. This problem has also been manifest in the VA geriatric-fellowship program where some positions have, to date, gone unfilled. Several strategies for overcoming this applicant famine can be suggested. Early marketing efforts of the training program must be aggressive, perhaps with better salaries offered than in more sought-after areas. An early priority should be the introduction of rotations of adequate length early in the core residencies of the primary-care specialties. Another should be the creation of the clinical and research experiences for students in the better geriatric units that are emerging nationally.

One problem faced by medical education in general that can be expected to be particularly acute in geriatrics is the difficulty that faculty have in accepting responsibility for creating an environment in which emerging graduates of new training programs can function appropriately. Historically, innovative undergraduate and graduate training programs have faltered because of the absence of the necessary environmental supports that would permit the graduates to function in settings appropriate to their training. Although we are quick to recognize that the role of environment in determining patterns of practice is as great as, if not greater than, that of training, the academic institution has been relatively reluctant to become actively involved in shaping that practice environment. As a result, the graduate has considerable difficulty in applying in practice the techniques he or she has mastered as a student. We are all too familiar with the paradigm of the academic training program that emphasizes complete evaluations of each patient treated. The resident trained to spend an hour in thorough investigation of each patient's problems suddenly becomes the practitioner with only thirty minutes to devote to each patient. Academic medicine is quick to label this community care as suboptimal but is much more reticent to develop the means to harness those thirty minutes most effectively. The bridge between academic and community practice will be a critical challenge in the area of geriatrics. There is a need to develop practical tools for everyday practice (for example, workable records systems and useful measures), as well as to undertake political efforts to gain professional recognition and to challenge stultifying government regulations affecting reimbursement.

9   Measurement Issues in Geriatrics

This chapter discusses measurement in geriatrics and its relationship to the education of geriatric personnel, especially medical personnel. The evaluation of any planning strategy directed at altering the health status of the elderly by changing the availability or skills of geriatric providers requires a technology for assessing that health status in the first place and detecting increments of progress. Efforts to train geriatricians or "gerontologized" practitioners require accurate and appropriate assessment tools that can be introduced through the educational process.

The subject is topical and complex. Assessment has become a buzzword in geriatric policymaking groups. A comprehensive, individualized assessment of the elderly person's functioning has been proposed as the open sesame for access to expanded long-term-care (LTC) benefits. Once services have been marshaled on behalf of the individual, program accountability also depends on regular assessment of the program recipient. Integral to this process is an ability to make accurate measurements of factors selected as important. Unfortunately, no agreement has yet been achieved on two of the most crucial points: (1) the identification of important factors to be measured, and (2) the technology for making these measurements.

Beyond a need for technical knowledge and skill derived from the medical subspecialties relevant for treatment of particular problems, those caring for the elderly require a general perception about the well-being of the older person that transcends a particular diagnosis, problem, or specialization. Many authorities have pointed out the limitations of a diagnosis-centered approach in viewing the health of the elderly (Kent, Kastenbaum, and Sherwood 1972; Sherwood 1975; Goran et al. 1976). Conventional wisdom now holds that (1) the elderly are subject to multiple diagnoses; (2) the physical, mental, and social well-being of an elderly individual are very closely interrelated, so that multidimensional assessments of health status are necessary; and (3) measures of functional status that examine the ability to function independently despite disease, physical and mental disability, and social deprivation are the most useful overall indicators to assist those caring for the elderly.

Where does this leave the physician or other health-care provider? The mandate for a global assessment of functioning presents a formidable and elusive task. The clinician needs practical tools that will permit evaluation of the individual's status, prediction of his or her future course, and planning for his or her care. In a way, measurements are organizers, capable of turning amorphous and expansive goals into a series of defined tasks. They are the means by which progress or lack of progress is noted. The bad image of geriatrics in the eye of neophyte physicians may be partly attributed to a perception that the patients are not amenable to change in status. To dispel such notions, physicians can be equipped with accurate and trustworthy techniques to help focus their attention on the positive changes that are indeed possible.

Who Makes Measurements in Long-Term Care?

The choice of measurements for use in long-term care depends on the role and purpose of the person making the measurements. At least four groups of measurers can be identified:

1. The physician (or substitutable health provider) who is not primarily a geriatric specialist but who encounters elderly persons in the course of an ambulatory or hospital practice.
2. The geriatric specialist.
3. The case manager.
4. The researcher and/or program evaluator.

The Nongeriatric Practitioner

As we have indicated already, physicians in their daily office and hospital practices encounter many patients over age 65 and even over age 75. In this context, the major purpose of a measurement of overall functioning would be as an aid to the physician in organizing observations and ensuring that no important factor is omitted from consideration. Brevity and practicality are key features. Estimating generously, the newly sensitized physician may spend a maximum of five extra minutes considering the functional status of his patient over and above the particular complaint under immediate care. Alternatively or additionally, other systematic information might be collected by office personnel or through a self-completed series of questions given to the patient. In either case, the most useful measurements will be those that can rather quickly help the provider assess the patient's total situation. As an outcome of such a measurement, the provider may turn attention to some problem amenable to medical assistance other than the one that brought the patient to him, or he may seek the consultation of a geriatric specialist.

As undergraduate medical educators seek to alert neophyte physicians to the complex needs of the geriatric patient and to resocialize such physicians into a more optimistic therapeutic stance toward the over-age-75 patient with multiple decrements in functioning, they will wish to equip new generations of physicians with convenient measuring tools that provide a frame of reference for treatment of their elderly patients. We might risk an analogy to the Apgar score for assessment of newborn children; although the score is recognized to be an accumulation of rather crude judgments, it has survived as a useful organizing tool with predictive validity. In the spirit of recognizing that one attends to what one can measure, and that the very act of measuring reminds the physician that more than one option for action is available, the search for appropriate brief measures for the nongeriatrician should be a priority.

Geriatric Specialists

Because the geriatric specialist will regularly treat the elderly person with multiple physical, psychological, and social problems, he will require a larger array of assessment tools than other physicians and will need to become proficient in measuring rather small distinctions in functioning. In geriatric-assessment units, such specialists will make recommendations for future care in intensive rehabilitation settings or in LTC institutions on the basis of the patient's total functional (physical, mental, and social) status and social supports. For the purposes of intensive rehabilitation, the specialist will want to note progress toward goals such as mobility, transfer, and other skills of self-care. In this chapter we will discuss some of the variations and refinements in existing functional-status measures. Informal discussions with geriatricians in Great Britain suggest that rate of change in functioning may be an important diagnostic and prognostic tool. The ability to educe measures of change rates is dependent on the ability to make repeated accurate measures in categories sufficiently fine to show change.

Practice in LTC institutions (or in community programs serving the same population that currently resides in nursing homes) will be enhanced if the geriatrician is able to measure differences at the lower end of the functional-status continuum. Although perhaps the majority of patients are coping with impairments of physical functioning, and many are impaired in their mental abilities as well, all chronic LTC patients cannot be lumped together and assigned an identical and gloomy prognosis (which all too readily becomes a self-fulfilling prophecy). A further consideration is the morale of the staff who work with the chronically impaired, often in institutional settings. They too, need to be shown how to observe small changes in functional abilities as a step toward encouraging them to be part of a team effort to promote the desired changes.

LTC institutions provide a drastic change of life-style for the residents. Ideally speaking, such changes are recommended for the protection, care, and ultimate well-being of the older person. Because the setting of care imposes new conditions on the patient's life, it is incumbent on the provider to be able to measure effects on subjective states of happiness, morale, or well-being and on objective states of social interaction and activity. Numerous technical problems arise in making such measurements, including (1) the selection of instruments or indicators; (2) the difficulty in making attribution to the institutional environment without baseline information about psychological and social well-being prior to admission; and (3) the difficulty in getting valid information because of the physical and mental disabilities of the patients and their dependence on caretakers.

Geriatricians cannot be expected to solve such measurement problems singlehandedly, nor is it likely that they will be the primary measurers of psychological and social well-being among the institutionalized elderly. In fact, some of this measurement falls under the rubric of program evaluation as discussed later, involving as it does group measures rather than measures focused on the individual resident. In terms of the individual patient, however, the clinician needs to be aware of the possibility of untoward effects of treatment and to develop a manageable way of noting them. If he has followed the patient through earlier phases of care, he may, with the right tools, be in a position to measure changes in psychological and social functioning over time and from pre- to postinstitutional life.

Case Management

The case manager is responsible for decisions about the way resources are allocated to an individual patient on the basis of the patient's need; the presumed effects of various management strategies on the patient's well-being; and, of course, the availability of resources across the total community. Case management as a formal function is just coming into its own in geriatrics. Field tests of case-management systems such as ACCESS and TRIAGE have been mounted with the assistance of waivers (U.S. Comptroller General 1979); these tests permit a more flexible use of funding available under Medicare and Medicaid. To a lesser extent, Professional Standards Review Organizations (PSROs) that have begun LTC review also engage in case management when they conduct a preadmission review to determine appropriateness of a nursing home for a patient; here, however, the PSROs are limited to the legalistic function of determining eligibility for funded services under the law rather than constructing ideal service packages.

The managerial function of the geriatrician has been emphasized in British literature (Anderson 1971; Brocklehurst 1978). Such a function implies that a package of services is created for a patient based on an individualized assessment of his needs and the likely benefit of services. A physician may not necessarily make all the assessments that lead to the service prescription, but it is argued that he serves as a coordinator. As formal case-management systems emerge in the United States as a means of controlling scarce resources, physicians may or may not be assigned the ultimate responsibility. Especially where public dollars are concerned, other personnel such as social workers, nurses, or some hybrid care provider yet to emerge may make the final choices. Nevertheless, physicians (or substitutable personnel) will always have an important role in case-management decisions and, in the private sector, may become de facto case managers, responsible for recommending a constellation of services to patients and their families.

What kind of measurement helps with case management? Here a composite measurement is required, constructed from an understanding of the functional status of the patient, his medical condition and prognosis, and his social resources. Value decisions about preferred modes of treatment (for example, a value for treatment in the least restrictive environment possible and for avoidance of institutional care) would affect the way scores on such a scale were used as guides to action. Although cutoff scores on such scales could hardly be used as a mechanical guide to a specific action, they can assist a case manager in reviewing the amount of care required by an individual, translating his functional limitations into practical factors relating to his capacity for self-care, considering the individual's affective state and social circumstances, and eventually reaching recommendations. Multidimensional assessment measures have also been used as tools to predict who will be able to remain in the community; to the extent that such scales have prognostic capability, they can be used to establish norms for the kinds and numbers of LTC services needed.

Case management does not cease of course, when a patient becomes a resident in an LTC facility. Then, too, a measure of overall functioning across a number of dimensions will suggest a plan for the care of that individual; as will be shown, however, the instruments used may differ from those used for community-based care management.

Research and Evaluation

In the first stage in enlightenment about geriatrics, the neophyte is usually exposed to the burgeoning geriatric literature. Here many assertions about aging and subgroups of elderly persons are encountered, along with discussion of the relative merits of various approaches in achieving goals (such as longevity, alleviation of depression, and improvement of functional status).

The literature is replete with correlational studies reporting the relationship of demographic and other variables with the health status of the elderly; much less frequently one also finds studies of cohorts of elderly persons over time. Such statements, although interesting to the geriatric specialist, cannot be evaluated without reference to the measurements on which the statements are based.

Recent reviews of measurements in long-term care (Bloom 1975) or of classes of measurement, such as measures of (1) functional status (Katz, Hedrick, and Henderson 1979), (2) subjective well-being or happiness (Larson 1978; George 1979, (3) life adjustment (Graney and Graney 1973), and (4) mental functioning or depression (Salzman et al. 1972; Raskin and Jarvik 1979), indicate that measurements are numerous but often not thoroughly tested. In some instances, measures that were developed on youthful populations or for specialized populations (such as psychiatric patients) are applied to the elderly. In other instances, investigators have chosen to develop yet another instrument rather than use one that had already been fielded with an older population.

As a general rule, the clinician will not be involved in methodological research designed to develop measures or in descriptive epidemiological studies of the aging process. Interface with the research-and-evaluation enterprise, however, occurs rather passively when the gerontological literature is read, and more actively when measures are sought to study the effects of a clinical treatment or a management intervention on the general functioning and well-being of the patient. Some portion of the geriatric specialists being trained for the future (especially those who will assume positions of leadership in teaching settings) will be engaged in clinical research and program evaluation. Choice of measurements determines the way in which reality is abstracted; the clinician cannot assume that all measures of concepts such as functional status, mental orientation, or adjustment really measure the same thing. In program evaluation, "measurement overkill" is an ever-present hazard because of the tendency to include a large number of scales and composite measures that yield scores as a substitute for careful targeting on ways to measure the desired outcomes of the program.

Figure 9-1 depicts the relationship of measurement to research and evaluation in long-term care. As the sequencing shows, the need to begin with characteristics that can be measured gives rise to a body of methodological research aimed primarily at ensuring the reliability and validity of the measurements themselves. Research should also be directed at showing how characteristics are correlated with each other and how they vary according to demographic or situational distinctions. A characteristic under scrutiny is conventionally dubbed an "outcome" if it is sought as a treatment goal or encountered as an untoward result of treatment. Descriptive studies and longitudinal research, so important in developing an under-

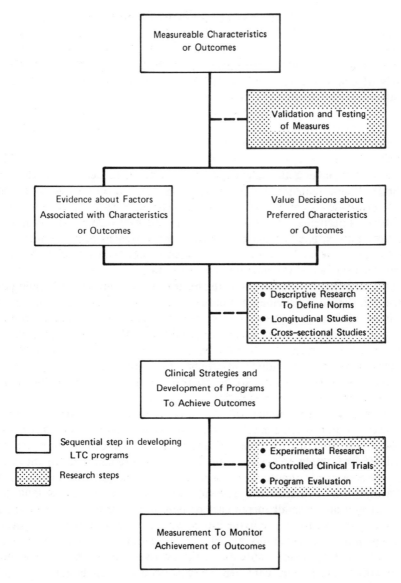

Figure 9-1. Schematic Representation of Relationship of Measurement to Research and Evaluation in Long-Term Care

standing of normal aging and establishing inferences about causality, are dependent on the adequacy of the measurements in the first place. The selection of clinical goals, however, does not depend on the body of research alone; it also depends on value decisions about the preferred results of treatment. Such values may be consciously defined and expressed, or implicit; they may reflect preferences of the provider community, those of the elderly person, or some societal synthesis. If one is armed with evidence about factors associated with aging and with value statements about the kinds of characteristics deemed desirable as program outcomes, clinical strategies can be developed and tested.

Group Versus Individual Measures

Criteria for judging the adequacy of an instrument depend in part on whether that instrument is being used to assess the status of an individual or to describe a group of people. In making a clinical determination about the health of a particular person on which one will base recommendations for that person's care, it is essential to strive for the greatest accuracy possible. In so doing one is likely to produce a large number of categorical distinctions growing out of the numerous possible variations on a human theme. On the other hand, estimations of the health status of groups of individuals are often needed to provide a groundwork for program decisions; such decisions could occur at the level of a single organization (such as an LTC center planning the differential expansion of programs and services) or on the level of a community, state, or larger region. In such instances, a large number of observations of each individual would be impractical and undesirable. Instead, one seeks a readily applicable instrument that suggests the extent and nature of need in the population.

The desirable attributes of individual measures are compared with those of group measures in table 9–1. Although the basic requirements for reliability and validity apply in both instances, our table shows some of the tradeoffs that might be made on the basis of the use intended for the data and the constraints imposed on data collection. In the case of the individual measures, we emphasize the detection of remediable problems and the documentation of small increments of change as a means of measuring progress. In the case of group measures, we are more concerned with problems of inter-rater reliability and the identification of practical measures that can be aggregated. This distinction between individual and group measures becomes irrelevant when the sums of individual-change scores are used rather than a comparison of group means. To make the distinctions clearer, we draw the extreme contrast between a measure used by a planner in a broad-population study and one used by a clinician planning the care of an individual elderly person. As later discussions show, the distinctions are not always so clear cut.

Whether the instrument is designed to measure individual or group

Table 9-1
Attributes Desired in Individual and Group Measures in Long-Term Care

Individual	*Group*

Reliability
  Across raters
  Over time
	Reliability
	  Across raters
	  Over time

Validity	Validity
Minimizing false negatives	Capability of producing useful broad categories of functional ability across the whole spectrum of performance
Minimizing false positives	
Capability of documenting problems amenable to intervention	Minimizing the time and cost of administration
Capability of documenting conditions requiring a service strategy	Minimizing the cost of analysis
Capability of documenting small changes in functioning	Portability—minimize equipment required
	Reproducibility across geographical and cultural lines
Defensible strategy for sampling the behaviors measured	Minimizing dependence on professional judgment or implicit criteria
	Defensible strategy for sampling from the population

health status, reliability and validity are common concerns. Reliability refers to the capability (in the absense of real change) of obtaining the same result with repeated measurements. Reliability is at particular risk when measures depend on raters' judgments. In long-term care, many of the measurements of functional status in common use are, in fact, the cumulative observations of a professional or paraprofessional rater. Some organizations have reported high reliability among raters even when the tool used calls for many judgments; such inter-rater reliability is achieved through intensive training. It may be a fallacy, however, to assume that instruments that were proven reliable when used at specialized centers for the study of aging will be reliable in the hands of other personnel in other programs. To the extent that an instrument calls for ratings based on explicit criteria using highly specific and observable categories, the inter-rater-reliability problem is minimized.

Inter-rater reliability (or the ability of the same rater to achieve the same result with repeated measurements) is a vexing issue in long-term care. Whether the test is self-completed or observer completed, stability in the measurement over time is sought. If real changes occur in the subject between the two measurements, however, a change in score should indeed occur. (The same point applies to tests of inter-rater reliability unless observations can be made simultaneously by several raters.) Conventional clinical wisdom asserts that the elderly fluctuate in their functional abilities (based partly on factors such as fatigue or acute illness). The difficulty lies in distinguising when a change in a score is a result of a real change in status and not merely an artifact of the testing situation. For example, some tests of cognitive ability can be learned, so that one might expect successive improvements on retest; others may become irritating to the respondent, so that one might expect a decrease of effort and cooperation. A catch 22 is presented: without reliable measurements, we cannot be certain about the extent of fluctuation in functional status, and we cannot readily test the measures for reliability without assuming some stability over time in the characteristic measured.

Validity, or the ability of a measure to reflect the characteristic it is intended to assess, is, of course, the ultimate aspiration of all measures; it is equally important whether the object of scrutiny is an individual elderly person or a population. Validity issues are discussed later in the context of particular attributes measured in long-term care (for example, activities of daily living, mental status, life satisfaction, social support); but some general comments can be made. Many of the qualities that are considered important outcomes of long-term care are highly abstract ones such as morale or independence. Little agreement exists among laypersons on the meaning of such terms, and there is a danger that instruments used to measure them will, in fact, measure only a limited aspect of what is commonly meant by the phenomenon. Worse, the measurement may be associated with an idiosyncratic definition of the concept that would not be shared by many others.

The validity of a particular data set is influenced by the internal characteristics of the measurements used, as well as by the administration of the instrument and the nature of the sampling. Obviously, a statement about the attributes of a group of elderly persons must be based on an adequate sampling technique to ensure representativeness and an information-collection strategy that does not bias the information received. The latter involves safeguards of confidentiality; creation of an environment permitting disclosure of feelings; and consideration of any particular limitations (hearing speech, physical frailty) of the respondents that might affect the results. Less obviously, sampling is an important issue even when a clinician is measuring the status of one individual patient or elderly person. Here the key decisions involve the sampling of observed behaviors, the time window used, and the frequency of observation that is incorporated into a measure.

The points of contrast between group and individual measures represent not absolute differences, but relative emphases. The community planner conducting a population study seeks an easily used instrument that, in turn, suggests a selfadministered questionnaire, an instrument amenable to group administration, or an instrument that can be personally administered in a fairly brief interview. Because volume is emphasized, an ideal instrument should not require a high level of professional education to administer; and it should lend itself to analysis with minimal intermediate steps. To preserve flexibility of administration, it is best that the instrument be independent of elaborate or expensive equipment. To preserve accuracy, it is best that the judgment of the raters be minimized. Such an instrument should be able to produce a manageable number of broad categories of ability across the full range of the expected performance spectrum. In developing general categories, however, it is probable that much specific information relating to a particular individual will be lost.

In contrast, a clinician will want to minimize both the false positives and false negatives associated with a measure. Precision, in terms of measuring the status of a particular individual, will probably be more important than ease and economy of administration, analysis, and interpretation. Protecting the time of professional personnel is also less relevant, particularly because those personnel will already be involved in a therapeutic and prescriptive sense. A functional-status measurement used in assessing impaired persons is sometimes needed to differentiate small changes at the lower end of the spectrum; this is particularly true in the case of stroke victims or mentally disoriented persons whose changes in status may be minute and slow. Further, a measurement should have some pragmatic application in the sense that it can document the problems and conditions that are most amenable to intervention and that would suggest a specific service strategy. Because an infinite amount of information could be collected about an elderly individual, it is important that decisions about what to measure and the cutoff points used have practical utility. The practitioner, however, must not lose sight of the importance that small distinctions in functional ability can have for the quality of life of the geriatric patient. For example, the strength to sit up, especially the ability to do so for several hours, makes an enormous difference to the patient. In another example, a small improvement in the patient's use of a hand may be the key to communication.

Purposes of Long-Term-Care Measurements

Examining LTC measures in a somewhat different way, the major function of an instrument should be considered. Table 9-2 separates five functions: description, screening, assessment, monitoring, and prediction. The major uses of each function and the characteristics of the desirable instrument are discussed in this section.

Table 9-2
Major Functions, Purposes, and Desirable Characteristics of Long-Term-Care Measurement Instruments

Function	Purposes	Characteristics
Description	Depict elderly population along selected parameters. Describe outcomes associated with various intervention forms. Develop normative data. Assess needs. Use as tool in hypothesis testing.	Reliability; face and construct validity.
Screening	Identify from among populations at risk those individuals who should receive further assessment	Reliability; easily administered, inexpensive measures of variables having practical significance; minimize false negatives.
Assessment	Diagnosis. Assignment to interventive strategies.	Reliability; face and construct validity. Detailed measures that clearly delineate functioning in small units; practical significance; accuracy (that is, minimizing both false positives and false negatives); sufficient sampling of items measured to minimize error.
Monitoring	Reviewing progress of those receiving treatment. Observing change in untreated condition.	Reliability; face and construct validity. Does not need to be as detailed as assessment tool. Time intervals between monitoring selected on basis of likely change. Consideration of cost, time and amenability to self-monitoring by patients.
Prediction	Make prognostic statements of expected outcomes on the basis of given conditions. Permit scientifically based clinical interventions. Add strength to case-management decisions.	Reliability of measurement. If a measurement predicts an outcome, it does not need to be tested for validity. Face validity, however, makes prediction more acceptable to users.

Description

Description is a basic function that permits establishment of a body of information about the elderly population along selected parameters. It is important to be able to describe the population as a whole in order to develop normative data and to assess needs. One also wants to record the outcomes associated with care and to test hypotheses about the effectiveness of various interventions. For all this descriptive work, a bank of well-validated, reliable measures is required.

Screening

Screening is another function of measurement that is often advocated. By its very definition, screening is not expected to be error free; rather, it should indicate the need for further intensive assessment. Ideally, a screening instrument should be practical and inexpensive; this is especially true if the population at risk is as large as is envisaged in discussions of screening for the elderly. (For example, it is sometimes suggested that all patients over 65 who are recently bereaved should be screened for depression or that all those over 75 should be periodically screened for their ability to cope, a composite measure of functional status balanced against social resources.) A screening instrument can rarely eliminate false positives and false negatives equally well. The relative merits of emphasizing one over the other will depend on the prevalence of the condition and the cost of further evaluation. At the screening level, minimizing false negatives would probably be best if, indeed, a helpful therapeutic or preventive intervention is available when further assessment indicates the need for services.

Assessment

Assessment involves a more detailed review than does screening and leads directly to diagnostic conclusions and assignment to interventive strategies. The terms *screening* and *assessment* are bandied about in the LTC field, often without any clear distinction between them. It may be that very few measures, especially in the psychosocial areas, are suitable for screening in long-term care, but rather that periodic assessment is necessary. Certainly LTC recipients are likely to change suddenly in important particulars. Although screening for some diseases and impairments (hypertension, glaucoma, hearing problems) could occur according to a fixed timetable with little likelihood of change between the intervals of measurement, the same assurance is not possible when screening for most physical, psychological, and social problems. In fact, screening, especially for psychosocial problems, might best be performed by examination of some very straightforward risk indicators (for example, recent bereavement as a risk factor for depression or social disruption) followed by a detailed assessment at the time of the first encounter with the individual at risk.

Assessment has become a keystone of geriatric practice. Each discipline claims its need to make particular assessments on the dimensions that concern it most. Psychosocial assessments, mental-status examinations, physical-therapy assessments, occupational-therapy assessments, social-work assessments, and drug-regimen reviews are terms that connote the lack of clarity over whether assessments take their particular definition from the content focus or from the discipline performing the evaluation. There is no disputing that the assessment of the geriatric patient (or, on a community basis, the assessment of needs of the elderly) must be multifaceted and multidisciplinary. Recording formats have been developed for nursing-home residents to facilitate an amalgamation of information systematically contributed from different disciplines. The best example of this is the Patient Appraisal and Care Evaluation (PACE) system developed by the Department of Health, Education, and Welfare (DHEW) for assessing nursing-home patients (U.S. DHEW 1978a, 1978b). Designed as a case-management tool for nursing-home residents, the system does not contain rules for how the assessment team can use the information to develop specific plans based on combinations of observable factors. Similarly, other multidimensional assessment tools have been developed that, although they may not require the literal involvement of an interdisciplinary team to collect the information, contain items that reflect functioning across many domains. In these cases, too, the multidimensional assessments often fail to provide a measure of overall functioning that takes into account the several dimensions. Assessment of need for services must be made on the basis of composite measurements; it may be that an indicator such as physical functioning, although crucially important in itself, bears little direct relationship to the amount of care required from community services or the decision about the locus of such care.

Monitoring

Monitoring involves repeated measurements to assess change in status. It may be undertaken as an adjunct to treatment or as an observation technique to note change over time in a particular condition of an untreated patient. Monitoring general functional status does not usually require the same detailed measurement as does initial assessment because parameters of expected change are specified. Cost and convenience are important factors; it is an advantage if patients can perform the monitoring themselves. Obvious examples of monitoring measures that can readily be performed by most patients are weighing themselves or taking their own blood pressure. Patients might also be taught to make important regular observations of functional-status dimensions such as mobility and falls or continence. As yet, the development of measures that can be readily used by patients and their families as monitoring devices has not received much attention; perhaps the ability of the elderly to participate in such functions has been underestimated.

Monitoring implies the importance of measuring change; therefore, the intervals between monitoring should be derived by some empirical notions of the rapidity of expected deterioration or improvement in the condition being monitored. Here we go back to the more basic measurement function:

description. Until normal aging under a variety of circumstances is better described, it is rather difficult to know how often to measure or when the rate of change has reached alarming proportions.

Prediction

The foregoing discussion leads to the last function of measurement, prediction. To some extent, all clinical treatment involves prediction. At least informally, the clinician acts on a prediction that a given form of intervention will produce a desirable result. For a measure to be used as a prognosticator, it must be reliable and well designed. Longitudinal studies using these measurements have shown that certain outcomes are consistenly associated with scores of the measures. Such studies may describe either the natural course of change in measurable attributes for categories of people or the change in measurable attributes associated with therapeutic intervention. If a measure can be used to predict an outcome, the association implies predictive validity. Nevertheless, if a measurement or a score has face validity (that is, if it makes common sense), practitioners are more willing to use it as a prognostics indicator. In long-term care, examples can be given of discriminant analyses that have revealed rather implausible factors that predict outcomes such as likelihood of discharge from nursing homes (Gutkin et al. 1979). As Sherwood and Feldman assert (1970), statistical predictions may complement clinical judgments even if they do not explain reasons for associations. Occasionally the statistical predictors fly in the face of practice wisdom. In such cases, it is especially necessary that the initial findings be reproduced in replication studies.

Except in conditions of extreme limitation of physical functioning (as with comatose patients, for example), predictions in one domain of functioning must take into account the influence of other domains. Although predictive capability in measurement would lend comforting assurance to the work of case managers, the necessary studies of the relationships among aspects of overall functioning have not yet been done to make detailed predictions feasible. Clinical experience suggests that a promising lead for improving our prognostic technology is to pursue measurement of change rates in status rather than simply descriptions of a condition at any given point in time.

What to Measure?

As many writers have pointed out, long-term care embraces the spectrum of medicosocial–psychological problems of persons aged 65 and older. An enormous number of variables are related to medical and physiological conditions; physical, intellectual, and psychological functioning, as well as social well-being, could conceivably be introduced into the routine measurement of the clinician. Such an expansive approach to measurement would have disadvantages, however. It would be expensive and time consuming and would impose a burden on patients; moreover, in the face of potential information overlap, the distinctions between the important and the trivial could well disappear.

An analogy to the health care of children might illustrate the problem. Clearly, one could collect voluminous information about the functioning of children over and above information about the particular complaint, symptom, or problem that brought them to medical attention. Much of the information about the functioning of the developing child can be and has been expressed in terms of scores on particular scales. Thus it is possible to measure intelligence, cognitive development along a range of factors, body perceptions, health knowledge, school performance, motor functioning, relationships with peers, relationships with parents and siblings, communicativeness, affective states, and so on. Nobody has seriously suggested that such an assessment, using standard instruments, scales, and data-collection classification schemes, be used as part of a general pediatric workup. Yet some of the gerontological literature does seem to call for an elaborate list of measurements of elderly patients who come into long-term care.

In measuring everything from sexual functioning to memory loss, from ability to do chores to church attendance, the LTC provider faces problems. First, few persons of any age wish to permit detailed and intrusive measures of their performance without perceiving clear relevance to their well-being. Practical and ethical problems are greater if the individuals being assessed are physically frail or intellectually unable to give consent to procedures. Additional practical and ethical problems are created if the measurement necessitates collecting information from persons collateral to the patient. Furthermore, an attempt to develop scales to measure every relevant concept in long-term care may impede the refinement of our measurement tools. The test of relevance in choosing items to measure is applicable to both the clinician and the researcher, although the latter may cast a somewhat wider net.

Once a scale is created to measure a complex and abstract quality (for example, socialization patterns, authoritarianism, perceptions of control over one's life, future orientation), some practitioners tend to reify the scores. They may forget that the name given to the scale is an arbitrary one based on what the inventor believes it to reflect. But naming something does not always make it so—a horse named "Speedster" can still come in last. In other words, the users of the information may forget that a judgment about say, "life satisfaction" was based on a pattern of response to a few questions; they may regard the score as an absolute indicator of life satisfaction, comparable to a balance-scale in measuring body weight.

Not all observation results in a measurement or score. When information on a particular item is collected systematically along a continuum, then a measurement could be said to have occurred. Classification systems that collect information on a range of items can contain a number of separate measurements but do not necessarily combine these measures in a predetermined way to form a score representing a higher level of abstraction. For example, many PSROs have begun collecting information on individual physical functioning (Kane, R.A. et al. 1979), in some instances modeling their data collection on a classification system developed at Harvard University (Jones McNitt, and McKnight 1974). Although no composite score is derived, each item of the classification scheme constitutes a measurement that could be tested for reliability and validity. In contrast, scales of functional status have been developed that merge observations on discrete items into an overall scale that is meant to describe physical functioning.

In medical practice, not all items included in a history or physical examination incorporated as part of a systematic record lend themselves to continuous classification (checklists and dichotomous variables are also recorded), and not all classification is combined in a multiple-item scale. Decisions about what to measure also involve decisions about the way items of information can best be combined; raising the level of abstraction embodied in a score increases convenience in management of disparate facts but adds risk of oversimplification and error.

In choosing what to measure, the clinician will first be concerned with those characteristics that he deliberately wishes to change and, secondarily, with those characteristics that may be altered as a result of long-term care. Because patient management requires decisions that will often greatly alter the life-style of the patient, and because, in the name of long-term care, a patient sometimes enters a total institution, the happiness or subjective well-being of that patient is often included in the array of long-term-care measures even though the primary reason for delivering care may be related to other goals, such as increasing life expectancy, minimizing discomfort, or improving the functional status of the patient. In contrast, acute care is perceived as a time-limited intervention that interrupts normal life activities; therefore, although one strives to deliver such care in a humane manner, the measurement of a person's happiness while under care is not a predominant concern. In long-term care, the treatment or care interventions may be life-long, forcing the clinician to ask whether the social and emotional costs of receiving care in the form offered justify the protection or prolongation of life. To develop some information about this disturbing line of thought, measurements of subjective well-being are necessary.

In deciding what should be measured beyond the physiological measures embodied in the laboratory or radiological tests appropriate to the medical problem, the clinician should consider the typical LTC patient. The multiple diagnoses of the elderly patient result in a number of very common problems, which may occur singly or in combination. The most common problems occurring in long-term care are immobility, falls, incontinence, and mental confusion. Stroke is an extremely common disorder, which may be accompanied by any of the sequelae just mentioned, as well as by severe communication difficulties. Hearing and vision defects, also common in old age, combine with social isolation, depression, and loss of social-support systems. Physical, psychological, and social deficits are typically interactive, so that it is difficult to distinguish what is causative; but it is clear that a spiral of exacerbations occurs. For example, the presenting picture of a mildly confused individual who walks with difficulty, has a hearing loss, is depressed, and lacks social contacts does not lend itself to unraveling whether the sensory deficits and immobility have caused the confusion or what part depression and dwindling social contacts play in the situation. This is the prototype of the patient who typically challenges the geriatrician; whatever measurements are taken should be targeted to the multiple disabling conditions of such patients and the limitations that these impose for independent daily life.

The companion volume to this book (Kane and Kane 1981) includes a review of instruments in a number of categories of measurement that are important to the LTC provider:

1. *Measures of physical function.* These measures are frequently divided into ability to perform tasks of daily living or self-care and ability to perform more complex instrumental tasks. A measure of physical functioning is perhaps the most important general measure required in long-term care.
2. *Measures of mental functioning.* These measures are often divided into measures of cognitive or intellectual abilities and those of mental-health status, particularly affective functioning. This type of measure is almost as important as the previous one because it relates to the common problems of the LTC patient.
3. *Measures of subjective well-being.* A variety of terms such as morale, life satisfaction, happiness, and adjustment are used to connote subjective well-being, which becomes a concern to the long-term-care provider because his ministrations tend to be continuous and intrusive.
4. *Measures of social functioning.* These measures include the extent and nature of family and social support, activity levels, and participation in satisfying human relationships.
5. *Multidimensional measures.* Although the preceding measurement categories have been presented separately, the distinctions among them often blur. At the lower level of functioning, the conceptual lines distinguishing mental abilities, appropriateness of social relationships, and

physical abilities are often unclear. Even at higher levels of functioning, motivation rather than capacity may be at the root of some limitation rendering categorization within a construct rather ambiguous. Many investigators have developed measures that tap several domains of functioning. Some are combined into a single functional-status score, whereas others yield distinct scores on each separate, but related, dimension of functioning.

6. *Need for services.* An increasingly practical problem is to design a service package to meet the needs of a particular individual or to assess community needs compared with available services to make program-planning decisions. Measurement instruments designed for this purpose not only link the various aspects of functional status into some equation expressing need but also attempt to add a time dimension in terms of the amount of care required by the individual that is not available through a natural support system.

Conclusion

In this chapter we have emphasized the ways in which general measurements of the functional status of the elderly assist the geriatric provider. The choice of specific measurements will depend in part on the role of the measurer ("gerontologized" provider, geriatric specialist, case manager, or researcher) and the function of the measurement (description, screening, assessment, monitoring, or prediction). Additionally, some measurements are more appropriate as a clinical tool to guide those giving care to individuals, and some are more appropriate for producing information about groups of persons that could be used for program planning.

In a companion volume (Kane and Kane 1981), we examine available instruments in six major areas (physical functioning, mental functioning, subjective well-being, social functioning, need for services, and composite measures) according to the issues raised in this chapter. The reader is referred to that book for a discussion of the problems involved in making reliable and valid measurements in each of these spheres and for recommendations of particular tools that might be used by the practitioner.

10 A Research Agenda

In this chapter we turn our attention to the research component of a geriatric training program with special emphasis on health-services research. We will not emphasize the need for basic biomedical and social research in aging because these topics are well covered elsewhere (IOM 1978; NIA 1979; Finch and Hayflick 1977; Birren and Schaie 1977; Binstock and Shanas 1976). A detailed discussion of health-services research is also beyond our scope. We view research in the context of this report as both a need and an opportunity. The need is illustrated by some of the difficulties that we had in developing the information on which to project geriatric manpower. The opportunity is one of refocusing multidisciplinary research toward the health problems and care needs of the elderly, with full participation of the medical component—an ingredient that too often has been lacking.

We do not propose to generate here an exhaustive list of relevant topics for investigation by geriatric scholars. The IOM report has proposed a research agenda sufficient to occupy a legion of biomedical and social researchers. Indeed, the studies of aging already completed swell the lists of references included in many recent compendia, and most such studies raise abundant questions that merit further research. Our attention to research in this report on geriatric manpower stems from three intersecting themes:

1. In the course of developing geriatric-manpower projections, we identified a number of important topics on which data were either unavailable or insufficient. Research is needed to fill these gaps.
2. If geriatrics is to grow as a practice field, it must establish and nurture mechanisms for developing new knowledge relevant to practice. Our present understanding of the illnesses and functional decrements related to aging and their amenability to treatment is rather rudimentary. Opportunities abound to assemble the information that would permit health-care providers to make more confident predictions about the effects of their ministrations on the physical, psychological, and social status of their patients.
3. If geriatrics is to become established as an academic discipline (and this is necessary in order to educate either geriatric specialists or generalist physicians who are sensitive to the particular needs of geriatric patients), it must be able to make a contribution to the development of

knowledge. Clarifying and demonstrating the nature of such contributions, and establishing the means by which neophyte geriatricians can acquire the research skills to make them, is the task of those wanting to place geriatrics in the academic medical-school hierarchy. The first cohorts of academic geriatricians in the United States have a major obligation to report examples of clinically relevant research.

Problems in Making Manpower Projections

In the course of our manpower-policy analysis, we found that critically needed data were either unavailable or untrustworthy. As a result, we were often forced to resort to crude estimates, occasionally little better than educated guesses. We had two general kinds of problems: (1) in describing what kinds of services are currently being delivered to various subgroups of elderly persons by what kinds of health-care providers; and (2) in making judgments about the effects of such services on the functional status of the patient. Both problems lead us to our research agenda, but the first also suggests deficits in the retrieval of information as a result of poor records and statistics and a lack of common terminology for events (such as an office visit).

Health-services research is in itself severely impeded by our inability to track either patients or providers through routine information sources. We had difficulty determining how many persons in a variety of health professions either had received training to work with the elderly or had specialized in caring for them in practice. It was not clear whether those who serve predominantly elderly persons are the same group as those who received the special age-related training.

Patients are even more difficult to track than providers. Occasionally local PSRO areas have developed systems to monitor the appropriateness of both the acute and the long-term care received by elderly persons under Medicare and Medicaid (Kane et al. 1979); but their data do not permit us to determine to what extent particular patients reenter institutional care, either hospitals or nursing homes, after being discharged to the community. The way that utilization of primary-care physicians interacts with utilization of hospitals and nursing homes is not known at all. Tracking long-term-care (LTC) patients is particularly complicated because such persons often relocate geographically at times of medical crisis.

The problem of inability to track LTC services and thus judge the effectiveness of changes in care packages is not a new one. The difficulties were well demonstrated by the deinstitutionalization of mental-hospital patients. By and large, state hospitals did not follow up their discharges or note their return to the hospital in any systematic way; community mental-health centers did not keep records of services rendered to hospital dischargees or their outcomes. This poignant example illustrates the problems of a poor information system. Although scores of commentators agree that the policy of deinstitutionalization was a dismal failure in terms of meeting human needs, little documentation is available about the types of patients who had need for services, the kinds of services they needed, the timing of those needs, or what services they actually did receive and why these were inadequate.

Geriatric research must learn from this experience. An early step is the establishment of a workable data base. We hover on the brink of new social changes affecting the delivery of long-term care. The mix of institutional and noninstitutional services to the elderly is destined to shift; a redirection of manpower is likely. Geriatricians will be able to comment meaningfully on the results of any such changes only if we are able to note patterns in the way individuals utilize the spectrum of care and to associate at least gross outcomes (mortality, longevity, institutionalization) with such utilization.

In conducting the analyses described in this book, the state of knowledge did not permit us to extrapolate manpower needs on the basis of the abilities of differently trained individuals to bring about the desired outcomes. The two major impediments to this course of action were lack of knowledge about how clinical interventions affect outcomes and lack of knowledge about how the elderly, their families, or society value the different potential outcomes that might be attributed to long-term care. In simpler words, today we are unable to specify universal statements as to either what we could achieve in geriatric care or what we should achieve.

Our proposed research agenda for geriatric departments grows at least in part from the problems discussed above. We now turn to a topic-by-topic discussion of research directions that could be taken. Included on our list are the following kinds of investigations: refinement of health-status measurements; studies of effectiveness of care (with iatrogenesis an important subtopic); clinical epidemiology to establish norms for a geriatric population; development of prognostic indicators; examination of value preferences that elderly groups would use in making health-related decisions; and health-services research designed to show how services are utilized, how important health-related decisions of elderly persons are made, and the cost effectiveness of different kinds of care.

Measures

A prerequisite to geriatric health-services research is refinement of the methods for assessing and measuring the status of elderly persons. In chapter 1, we described the goals of a geriatric program in terms such as physical status, mental status, functional status, comfort, morale, independence, and appropriate longevity. In chapter 9, we discussed the problems involved in identifying useful measurements for operationalizing any of these goals in long-term care. It follows that work in developing measures must proceed if we are to ascertain our progress toward these goals.

In some cases, scales and measurement systems have been developed, validated, and proved reliable by widespread use in psychological and other experimentation. These need only be adapted for geriatric use. In most instances, however, measurement techniques need to be refined or new measures developed. Such work requires that each component be evaluated and that the entire instrument then be tested for accuracy, validity, reproducibility, and reliability.

The development of measurements requires the participation of psychometricians; such personnel may need to be attached to geriatric units so that the developmental work can proceed within the context of LTC delivery. Although physicians would not be expected to bear the brunt of this initial work, they will have important contributions to make. As already argued in an earlier chapter, the evaluation of program impact requires these tools; so, too, do clinicians monitoring the outcomes of their treatment. Furthermore, before the interaction of physical, mental, and social outcomes can be studied, each construct must be amenable to separate measurement.

Effectiveness of Care

Once measurement capability has been established, geriatricians can begin to examine the effectiveness of treatment. The effects of clinical regimens and of various patterns of care delivery can then be studied. The investigators would have the opportunity to show empirically to what extent the overall goals of long-term care (for example, survival, independence, contentment, freedom from discomfort, mental alertness) are compatible with each other and to what extent tradeoffs among goals are necessary.

The other side of effectiveness is iatrogenesis, and this too requires investigation. Because the elderly require a disproportionate amount of diagnosis and treatment, one would expect them to be vulnerable to a commensurate number of iatrogenic complications. Quantitative and qualitative assessment of the contribution of medical iatrogenesis to the disabilities of the elderly is an important research topic. We need to know to what extent medical interventions lead to a worsening of patients' conditions. In test populations, stratified to encompass common diagnoses and a wide range of functional status, one could assess what fraction of episodes of relatively sudden decline in health status are primarily or secondarily associated with medical procedures (such as drugs, treatments, or surgery). One could also assess the risk-benefit ratio for therapy, a parameter at least considered in younger persons, but rarely in the elderly.

Although medical interventions for the elderly are assumed to be fraught with danger (adverse drug reactions, for example, occur more frequently than in younger people), it is uncertain whether these reactions are due to inherent susceptibility or to poor compliance (perhaps produced by a combination of decreased memory and complex regimens). A useful series of studies could be designed to determine whether medical iatrogenesis is a major or a minor element in the overall health picture of the elderly and what proportion of it is attributable to patterns of care or other provider characteristics. Models for experiments in related areas are available to aid in the design of such studies (Jick 1977).

A more subtle dimension of the iatrogenesis question concerns the effects of the general patient-management decisions made by geriatric providers. Elderly persons have been known to manifest marked losses in functional ability, including declines in mental status, when moved to an unfamiliar environment. Seligman (1975) has termed this phenomenon of withdrawal and apathy among institutionalized individuals "learned helplessness." Disorientation is likely to be greater in unfamiliar surroundings. Rigid routines may leave the patient with aggressive, sometimes even abusive, behavior as the only available means of self-expression. If referral to a nursing home is made as part of a recuperative process, then this, as well as the drug or surgical procedure under study, might contribute to functional decline. This emotionally charged issue is susceptible to dispassionate objective study.

Clinical Epidemiology

Many of the issues relevant to geriatric practice can be approached from an epidemiologic perspective. We might begin with some very basic questions. For example, what are the problems that account for most of the hospital admissions among the elderly or for most of the LTC days? Such questions are not readily answered, and the answer to each part of this question may be quite different. Unfortunately, neither answer is likely to be readily available from the medical record. Such a comment is not a criticism of recordkeeping, but simply a recognition that most clinicians do not carefully identify precipitating events. For example, rarely does the clinician note the factors surrounding the fall that led to a fractured hip.

The cursory data available suggest that a few common problems account for a substantial proportion of the difficulties. For example, the most frequent causes for admission to geriatric wards in Britain are falls, strokes, incontinence, and mental confusion (Isaacs, Livingstone, and Neville 1972). These causes present us with multiple research opportunities in both clinical research and health-services research. The clinical researcher might study cardiac arrhythmias that affect cerebral blood flow or explore problems in proprioception and balance. The health-services researcher might investigate how the organization of services and the service-delivery environment exacerbate or ameliorate these problems. We have already noted the likelihood that many treatments and procedures are unnecessary. Similarly, the routines of the short-stay hospital may need altering for the elderly. If a geriatric patient spends three weeks without being dressed and allowed out of bed, the effects on functional abilities could be grave. As these examples suggest, geriatricians need to develop information about social and environmental factors correlated with the incidence and prevalence of common geriatric problems.

Research into these common problems of geriatrics offers an opportunity to combine the interests of the clinician and of the health-services researcher. For example, who is at risk from falls (or incontinence)? What are the circumstances associated with these untoward events in terms of physiologic phenomena (such as arrhythmias or hypertension in the case of falls), activities, and precipitating events? How effective is the therapy intended to rehabilitate those who fall (such as physical therapy)? Settings such as the VA offer an excellent opportunity for this type of research, although it is limited in generalizability by the special male population served. Because of the large identifiable and traceable population of VA hospitals, prospective studies can be considered. Long-term follow-up is quite feasible, thus permitting analysis of patterns of recurrence and comparison of treatment goals with actual outcomes. Treated groups can be compared with untreated or alternatively treated controls.

Imagination in the design of the environment of LTC patients and their routines may pay great dividends. Architectural design can provide ready availability of toilets to lessen incontinence. Reminders can often prevent soiling. Once again, more quantitative data on the relative efficiency of a unit designed and staffed to help patients function most effectively would be useful. Can such a unit save more than its marginal cost by reducing length of stay, using fewer and less-trained staff, and reducing staff turnover?

Toward Prognostic Indicators

Once outcome measures are clearly established, controlled clinical trials of various methods of managing elderly patients can be fielded and the effects measured in terms of physical, mental, and social functioning. Such trials are appropriate when genuine doubt exists about the relative merits of alternative approaches to an end that is clearly valued by the patient population. It is worthwhile, for example, to test the ability of geriatric-assessment units to maximize the patient's possibility of returning to the community or the extent to which geriatric day-hospital attendance is associated with improved functional status. For studies such as these, randomized assignment to various experimental (and control) conditions is both sorely needed and ethically justified when (1) resources are scarce so that there are more candidates for geriatric-assessment units or day hospitals than could presently be served, and (2) the effects of the care are uncertain. If care in specialized geriatric units was associated with decreased independence or well-being, one would not wish to proliferate their development. If, on the other hand, the services were beneficial, their expansion would be warranted. Similarly, controlled clinical trials can be used to test the marginal benefits of increments of service, for example, adding home visits of occupational therapists or adding counseling services.

Many times, however, controlled clinical trials are not appropriate for ethical or logistic reasons. Then the effect of services can be judged only in comparison with some reasonable prognosis of outcome for the particular case. This suggests a line of research directed at establishing average prognoses for conditions common to the elderly. (Although this technique is applicable to chronic disease in general, it has special relevance for the elderly, where advanced age may be an important factor to consider.) Prognoses for long-term-care patients with varying conditions must be established along the dimensions of all the important goals of geriatric care. Such work is a laborious but inescapable methodologic requirement for further studies of the elderly because it provides a basis for comparing outcomes of alternative treatment when randomized trials are not feasible.

In brief, elderly patients must first be classified according to a well-organized system of diagnosis and staging. Then a team of experts could make prognostic estimations related to goals of care, using temporal targets (such as three months, six months, or one year). The actual health status of each patient can be determined at each agreed-on point and compared with the original prognosis. Ultimately, when a set of reliable prognoses has been determined, these can be recorded and codified. Mathematical modeling can be used to identify those factors most useful in prediction. Such a process would be repeated until a sufficiently high level of predictive accuracy is achieved. The goal is to reduce such predictions to average prognosis statements, which can be applied to various populations with defined characteristics. Numerous iterations are needed to produce workable formulas for estimating such averages.

The result of these efforts is equivalent to a natural history for a group of patients with specified characteristics. This information provides a probability estimate of the role of change from one status to another, an estimate that offers a critical contribution to any efforts to describe decision trees for patient care (Kane and Kane, 1981).

Once available, average prognoses have ready application to many studies. For example, they can be used to determine whether monetary or other incentives to caretakers can lead to better outcomes than the standard prognoses. Another use would be to compare the cost and effectiveness of various configurations of health-care personnel. Two existing studies have indicated that geriatric nurse practitioners working with a physician can provide satisfactory primary care in nursing homes (Kane et al. 1976a; Mark et al. 1976). In one of these studies, a social worker also made a significant contribution to the outcome (Kane et al. 1976a). In neither study, however, were medical, psychological, or functional outcomes estimated and compared with those for a suitable control population of known average prognosis. Patients were not classified according to levels of necessary care, nor were several permutations of team health care assessed. Thus much remains to be done before these crucial questions can be answered. A manpower-policy analysis such as ours would be able to reach far more definitive conclusions if such studies had already been performed.

Similarly, studies are needed comparing effectiveness and cost of various configurations of living conditions and health-care settings. Alternatives to nursing-home placement (such as home-care plans, home-care-plus-day-care centers, or residential communities with specialized services available) are often suggested. The literature contains hints, however, that such plans may indeed be significantly more expensive than nursing-home care (Weissert et al. 1978). Whether they are correspondingly more effective than nursing-home care is not clear. We could rephrase this question to ask whether the average outcome is better than standard prognoses for patients at various levels of initial status. The experimental design needed to address such questions is self-explanatory.

A major development in the field of long-term care is the growing emphasis on case management. Data from the Government Accounting Office study in Cleveland have suggested that it is possible to classify both the care needed by and the services rendered to a population of elderly individuals. These can then be combined in a matrix. Further analyses can calculate the rate of change over time that can, in turn, be related to the care received (U.S Comptroller General 1977; Maddox and Dellinger 1978). This study utilized a taxonomy of services rendered that encompassed a wide variety of medical and social services. Longer periods of follow-up would permit more precise calculations of the probabilities of an elderly individual's going from one status to another.

Community-based programs have been funded on a demonstration basis to test the benefits of a comprehensive assessment as a basis for patient placement in settings other than the nursing home. Two of the best known programs—ACCESS in Rochester, New York, and TRIAGE in Connecticut—combine the assessment and placement functions with recurrent monitoring to assess the appropriateness of such placements. Again, questions could be phrased in terms of comparing the average outcomes with standard prognoses.

Value Preferences

Controlled clinical trials and comparisons against standard prognoses will help inform us about the effects of interventions. But such studies do not tell us what effects are desirable. For this information, another line of inquiry is needed into the health outcomes that are most valued by elderly persons. If an older person were to understand fully the risks inherent in each choice of therapy, what would his or her choice be? How risk aversive are the elderly? Which risks are most feared? Models for these kinds of explorations are provided by work in other fields, such as McNeil's studies of the choices of cancer patients for surgery or other therapies (McNeil, Weichselbaum, and Pauker 1978). Investigations of the choices of the elderly should extend beyond questions of regimens and medical procedures to issues of locus of treatment and the amount of life change the individual is willing to trade for increased life expectancy or for improved functional status.

Value preferences of family members and of taxpayers are also relevant to the kind of care that elderly persons seek or that is financed publicly. In the context of the geriatric unit, studies of the values of family members could also be undertaken. Here the questions would concern the degree to which independence of an elderly relative is valued above the safety or security of that individual and the family's convenience or peace of mind. It is not always clear that family members are aware of the likely implications of alternative choices when they make their decisions.

Furthermore, elderly persons and their families often make extremely important health-related decisions under enormous personal stress. Research into the correlates of decisions to undertake high-risk surgery, to enter a nursing home, or to move to another city for health reasons would be very useful. The role of family influences and social and economic circumstances in shaping such decisions also merits study (Kane 1978). Such information could help caregivers create conditions that will minimize the decisions of elderly people and their families to accept long-term care under conditions that they later regret.

Longitudinal Studies

A number of the studies mentioned in this chapter and elsewhere in this book refer to the need for measurements of change over time in a defined population sample. Longitudinal studies of the elderly have been a mainstay of gerontologic epidemiology for several decades. Although such studies may offer a rich data base on physiologic, biochemical, and social changes associated with aging, much less is known about the factors that relate various forms of treatment to changes in health status.

Prospective studies that begin with aging cohorts could provide much useful data on the natural history of changes in status and use of services and institutions. Studies such as the Duke Longitudinal Study provide useful models of how one can acquire important data on such questions as rates of institutionalization (Palmore 1970, 1974). The use of the broader population study of Alameda County in California illustrates the ways in which subpopulations of the aged can be extracted and followed as a distinct cohort to provide similar information (Vincente, Wiley, and Carrington 1979). The next step is to apply epidemiologic techniques to relate underlying problems and various patterns of services used to these changes in status, as was done in the Cleveland GAO study noted previously.

Clearly, no single population will suffice to answer all questions. Appropriate groups must be followed if one is to address rather specific questions of interest. To the degree that we can identify those factors that place a segment of the elderly at risk of developing the condition of interest, we can design more efficient longitudinal studies; but at the same time, a certain number of broadly based studies may be the best sources of data on which to formulate these concepts of risk.

Only a few geriatric programs will be able to muster the resources necessary to mount and maintain large longitudinal studies. However, most programs should be capable of conducting prospective studies of specific clinical entities where the groups at risk may be either elderly persons likely to be afflicted (to study causation) or elderly persons already afflicted (to study treatment).

Implementation

The foregoing has offered a sampling of the kinds of research that might be appropriate and feasible within an academic geriatric program. Such studies would call for multidisciplinary involvement, but the special knowledge of the physician would be a central ingredient. Studies range from laboratory investigations of the aging organism (not discussed here) to health-services research directed at providing an understanding of the impact of alternative service models. In between are a host of clinically relevant studies directed toward clarifying the imperfectly understood pathophysiological problems that plague the elderly.

Some of the studies undertaken in geriatric units in England provide examples of how asking "simple questions" can lead to complicated searches for answers. For example, the investigation of why old people fall necessitated raising the corollary question: Why do old people not fall? In turn, this led to a complex series of studies now in progress to illuminate the nature of gait and related stability and instability. Such studies are intellectually satisfying to investigators and are intriguing to students and potential recruits to the specialty.

Teamwork is required for many of the departures suggested in this chapter. In some instances, the geriatrician would need to reach out to colleagues in other medical-school departments, collaborating, for example, with urologists, orthopedic surgeons, biochemists, and psychiatrists. Other disciplines such as dentistry, pharmacy, and physical therapy are also clearly relevant. Such collaborative arrangements, especially with other physicians, help to establish the credibility of the geriatrics unit within the academic medical center.

Many of the research suggestions reviewed here obviously call for the involvement of social scientists of various kinds. Geriatric providers should be able to take advantage of the growing number of social scientists trained in gerontology. Gerontology centers have relatively recently turned their attention to those among the elderly who are frail and disabled. Current federal initiatives encourage the fruitful collaboration of medical and social science to meet the needs of the neediest of the elderly. The time is therefore ripe for creating an alliance between medical and social-science research in a clinical-geriatrics department.

11 Conclusions and Recommendations

This report has provided some guidelines with which to frame discussions of the needs for geriatric manpower. These discussions include consideration of both the number of geriatricians needed and some alternative configurations by which medical services to the elderly could be offered. Several lines of conclusions and recommendations flow from these considerations:

We favor a version of geriatric practice in which the geriatrician will provide some primary care in addition to serving as a consultant. Assuming a target of improved care for patients aged 75 and older, we estimate that by 1990 this country will require the equivalent of 7,000 to 10,000 geriatricians to fill these roles and to meet the need for academic geriatricians, if moderate use is made of nonphysicians. A useful midrange estimate would be 8,000 geriatricians.

Current levels of effort to produce geriatric manpower will not produce sufficient supplies to meet projected needs for either academics or practitioners. A gradualist strategy for geriatric training seems the more reasonable course as opposed to a massive bolus effort. Efforts are needed to increase both the training opportunities and the pool of trainees. More programs are needed to train geriatricians and other health personnel in geriatrics; but the additional postgraduate positions will not attract enough good candidates unless additional steps are taken to make a career in geriatrics attractive. Various steps can be recommended:

1. Undergraduate programs in geriatrics must be created where they do not now exist and augmented where they do. Geriatrics and gerontology should be incorporated into the body of medical and health-professional education. We might offer subsidized clerkship experiences similar to the Public Health Service's Commissioned Officer Student Training and Education Program (COSTEP), where students assigned to preceptor-staffed clerkships can see first hand what is involved in the delivery of care to aged populations.
2. We need to expand both the number and quality of geriatric fellowships to provide exciting opportunities for intensive training in geriatric medicine for those who have completed core residency training in a variety of fields, including internal medicine, family practice, psychiatry, and neurology. These fellowships will need to compete successfully with those offered by other subspecialties. Recognizing the ubiquity of

ageism among young physicians, efforts should be directed toward developing inducements for entering geriatric training. This might include offering higher training stipends, identifying research opportunities and providing appropriate training, and increasing recognition and psychological support.

3. Geriatric role models are necessary both in practice and in academic settings. We have already indicated our support of the scenario that includes geriatricians in both of these settings. Students will not be stimulated to consider careers in a field unless they have some direct notion of what such an activity is like.

4. The prestige of geriatrics must be increased. This step impinges on several areas:

    a. Professional societies must be strengthened in both their practice and academic membership.

    b. Geriatrics must receive greater academic recognition. Faculty working in this field must be viewed as worthy of promotion and of full membership in the academic community. Teaching time must be given over to subjects germane to aging and the care of the elderly (although separate courses may not be necessary or desirable). Highly visible units (preferably divisions or sections within existing clinical departments rather than autonomous departments) should be formed in each medical school.

    c. Some means of professional recognition must be given to advanced training in geriatrics. Although we have not advocated specialty status per se, some form of certification is necessary.

5. Payment schemes for medical practice should be altered from the current procedure-oriented mechanisms to recompense time spent in personal care more equitably.

6. Mechanisms for the accreditation of training programs in geriatrics must be established.

Because primary-care physicians will continue their responsibility for much of the care of the aged, geriatrics must become a substantial part of their postgraduate training. This responsibility emphasizes as well the need for more geriatric content in undergraduate medical education.

A cadre of geriatric nurse practitioners (GNPs) and physician's assistants (PAs) will greatly aid in meeting manpower needs. More training programs to produce GNPs are needed, but training is not enough. In order to function appropriately, a GNP must practice in a supportive environment. Two major blocks must be removed:

1. Regulations must be changed to allow GNPs to prescribe under a limited formulary.

2. Medicare regulations must be amended to allow direct payment for GNP services remote from a physician supervisor if GNPs are to serve populations in great need, such as those in nursing homes.

Academic geriatrics must be encouraged in nursing schools as well as in medical schools. An academic path for the GNP is necessary if we are to have nursing faculty with clinical expertise and experience. Doctoral programs to offer such individuals research expertise are essential if GNPs are to enter the academic track and proceed successfully; these doctoral programs are located within the university health-sciences center.

Although there is growing support for biomedical research related to aging, we need more support for health-services research on improving services delivered to the elderly. In particular, we need to develop and test innovative modes of health care for the aged, including the substitution of social for medical services.

We require basic data on the quality and quantity of all types of health-care personnel available and needed for geriatric care.

We should adopt a standardized set of measures and vocabulary with regard to the care of the elderly. Although more work is needed to develop new and better measures of health (in its broader sense), current measures abound. The lack of standardized measures severely impedes the comparison of results from different studies. One dramatic example of the lack of common vocabulary is the varying definition of the group labeled "the aged." For example, most statistics deal with those 65 and older; most geriatricians focus on those over age 75, but some gerontology programs begin with persons as young as 55 or 60.

Appendix A: "Is Anybody Listening?"

'Is Anybody Listening?'

The following letter was forwarded to The Times by the author's niece. Neither woman identified herself "because we are fearful." Although The Times ordinarily will not accept anonymous articles for publication, the editors believe that this woman's message is exceptional.

Hello! Is there anyone out there who will listen to me?

How can I convince you that I am a prisoner?

For the past five years, I have not seen a park or the ocean or even just a few feet of grass.

I am an 84-year-old woman, and the only crime which I have committed is that I have an illness which is called chronic. I have severe arthritis and about five years ago I broke my hip. While I was recuperating in the hospital, I realized that I would need extra help at home. But there was no one. My son died 35 years ago, my husband, 25 years ago. I have a few nieces and nephews who come by to visit once in a while, but I couldn't ask them to take me in, and the few friends I still have are just getting by, themselves. So I wound up at a convalescent hospital in the middle of Los Angeles.

All kinds of people are thrown together here. I sit and watch, day after day. As I look around this room, I see the pathetic ones (maybe the lucky ones—who knows?) who have lost their minds, and the poor souls who should be out but nobody comes to get them, and the sick ones who are in pain. We are all locked up together.

I have been keeping in touch with the world through the newspaper, my one great luxury. For the last few years I have been reading about the changes in Medicare regulations. All I can see from these improvements is that nurses spend more time writing. For, after all, how do you regulate caring?

Most of the nurse's aides who work here are from other countries. Even those who can speak English don't have much in common with us. So they hurry to get their work done as quickly as possible. There are a few caring people who work here, but there are so many of us who are needy for that kind of honest attention.

A doctor comes to see me once a month. He spends approximately three to five seconds with me and then a few more minutes writing in the chart or joking with the nurses. (My own doctor doesn't come to convalescent hospitals, so I had to take this one.) I sometimes wonder about how the nurses' aides feel when they work so hard for so little money and then see that the person who spends so little time is the one who is paid the most.

I notice that most of the physicians who come here don't even pay attention to things like whether their patient's fingernails are trimmed or whether their body is foul-smelling. Last week when the doctor came to see me, I hadn't had a bath in 10 days because the nurse's aide took too long on her coffee break. She wrote in the chart that she gave me a shower—anyway, who would check or care? I would be labeled as a complainer or losing my memory, and that would be worse.

It is now 8 o'clock. Time to be in bed. I live through each night—and it is a long night—with memories of my childhood. I lived on an apple farm in Washington.

I remember how I used to bake, pies and cakes and cookies for friends and neighbors and their children. In the five years I have been here, I have had no choice—no choice of when I want to eat or what I want to eat. It has been so long since I have tasted fruit like mango or cherries.

As I write this, I keep wishing I were exaggerating.

These last five years feel like the last five hundred of my life.

Last year, one of the volunteers here read us a poem. It was by Robert Browning. I think it was called "Rabbi Ben Ezra." It went something like this: "Grow old along with me, the best of life is yet to be." How can I begin to tell you that growing old in America is for me an unbelievable, lonely nightmare?

I am writing this because many of you may live to be old like me, and by then it will be too late. You, too, will be stuck here and wonder why nothing is being done, and you, too, will wonder if there is any justice in life. Right now, I pray every night that I may die in my sleep and get this nightmare of what someone has called life over with, if it means living in this prison day after day.

□

Published in the *Los Angeles Times*, September 23, 1979 (anonymous). Copyright 1979, *Los Angeles Times*. Reprinted by permission.

Appendix B:
Methods for Calculating
Numbers of Practicing
Geriatricians Needed

The Concept of Need

Economists dislike the term "need" because it implies that needed services are desirable whatever the cost in other goods or services. However, if services are cheap or easy to get, people choose to get more than their needs; and if they are expensive or difficult to get, then people may substitute a less desirable alternative or even go without. In the medical field, "needs"— expressed in terms such as numbers of beds per capita, doctor/patient ratios, or visits for a given condition—vary widely from area to area and over time.

In theory, one good method for gauging needs would be to look at the effects of the "needed" resources on health. It is important in such an examination to distinguish the marginal effect of the last unit of the resource on health from the all-or-nothing total effect. For many interventions, there are sharply decreasing marginal returns; that is, some care is very helpful, but more care is unimportant. For example, whereas it apparently makes a considerable difference for infant mortality whether the mother sees a doctor once before delivery, there is little difference between some care and "adequate" prenatal care, once other demographic and economic factors are controlled for (Shah and Abbey 1969). A similar example is the frequency of cancer screening—semiannual Pap smears have little marginal advantage over annual ones (Eddy 1979).

Unfortunately for our purposes, we do not know the effects of various levels of medical personnel on the health of the elderly, and must therefore rely on expert opinion or current utilization. The problem with expert opinion, as reflected in professional standards, is that professional organizations have the incentive to set standards of care higher than the point of diminishing returns. For example, they may argue that a particular procedure should be done only by persons with a specified level of training, instead of examining the competence of those wishing to perform the task. The result might be a projected need for more highly trained persons than would necessarily be the case.

Projections based on current utilization are flawed by the assumptions that the current provision of services is good and that the pattern will remain stable over time. The economic theorems that show the optimality of market equilibria rely on assumptions that do not apply in the health-care sector—namely, the competitiveness of the supplying market, adequate information and access by the consumer, and payments by those obtaining the benefits. Using demand implies that currently underserved groups will remain so. Insofar as the health-care sector is able to generate its own demand, utilization is shaped to fit the desires of the providers rather than those of the consumers.

The standard evidence supporting the creation of demand includes the ability of hospitals to maintain occupancy after new construction (Roemer 1960), the association between the number of operations in the country and the number of surgeons (Bunker 1970), and the differential rates of hospitalization in fee-for-service and prepaid health-care systems (Klarman 1969). Later in this appendix we investigate whether utilization by the elderly appears to be high or low relative to that by younger groups after controlling for illness, but this does not tell us whether the higher or the lower utilizing group is getting the appropriate level of utilization.

Critics of the use of utilization data as the source for projections frequently point out its propensity to preserve patterns of maldistribution. This liability is not grievous for our purposes because we are concerned with estimating overall manpower requirements for a subgroup rather than local-area requirements. Moreover, we can modify our projections by inflating these estimates to approximate conditions when need would appear to be more fully met. The figures derived through such a process should suffice for general discussions about the magnitudes of manpower needed.

Our strategy for making this adjustment was to take utilization by middle-aged groups as our criterion for adequate care. We applied this approach to two different measures of utilization. Because the elderly have worse health in terms of a host of measures, we have used multivariate analysis to investigate the effects of these health measures on utilization. We then compared the utilization by the elderly with that of the middle aged, after controlling for health, and took the discrepancy as one component of unmet need. In addition, from the analysis described in chapter 2, we noted that physician time spent per visit, in both hospital and nonhospital settings, declines systematically with the age of the patient. We took as unmet need the difference between time per visit spent on those 45 to 54 and time per visit spent on the elderly, controlling for location, provider type, severity of condition, and episode type.

Are the elderly underserved relative to others? Utilization of hospital days and doctor visits is higher for the elderly than for younger groups. However, the health of the elderly—in terms of numbers of chronic conditions, limitations of activity, and self-restricted activity days, as well as perceived health status—is also worse. Perhaps if need is taken into account, they are actually getting less care.

To test whether the elderly are getting more or less care, we used a multivariate regression of utilization based on the National Health Interview Study (NHIS) data comparing those over 65 with members of a younger age group. The choice of the younger group was made to balance two considerations. We wanted the younger group to be comparable in terms of health, but different in whatever factors might affect access—money, mobility, or desirability as patients to a doctor. We selected all persons from 55 to 59 as the younger group and compared them with all those surveyed who were 65 years and older. The raw figures on health status and health-care utilization are shown in table B-1.

Note that there are two sets of estimates for doctors' visits. The NHIS asked respondents for the number of doctor visits in the preceding two weeks, and also in the preceding twelve months. Using the preceding two weeks reduces recall error but greatly reduces the effective sample size because only about 15 percent will have had doctor visits in that time period. For overall population estimates, the error from using the two-week recall is tolerable. For example, for people aged 65 or over, the estimate is 6.8 visits per year; the relative standard error of this estimate is only 2.5 percent (U.S. DHEW 1976). For smaller subgroups, the error can be much larger. For people over age 85, for example, the estimate is 6.2 visits per year, but the relative standard error is 15 percent. Using the twelve-month recall period adds recall error (generally forgetting) but greatly increases the number of events in the sample. Thus the average number of visits recalled

Table B-1
Measures of Health and Health-Care Utilization According to Age, United States, 1976

Health Measure	Age					
	55–59	65–69	70–74	75–79	80–84	85 +
Number chronic conditions	0.41	0.60	40	0.78	0.86	1.09
Restricted-activity days[a]	28	35	40	40	47	53
Percentage with some limitation of activity	27	39	43	49	54	64
Percentage who feel their health is fair or poor	24	32	31	32	31	32
Hospital days per year	1.6	2.4	2.7	3.0	3.4	3.9
Doctors visits[a]	6.2	6.4	7.5	6.5	7.6	6.2
Doctor visits (based on annual recall)	4.9	5.1	5.9	5.9	5.9	5.9

Source: Rand analysis of the National Health Interview Survey data (1976).

[a] Per year based on two-week recall.

in the preceding year is 5.6, about 80 percent of those that may actually have occurred.

Because most people estimate visits by counting those they remember, this downward bias is to be expected. The variability (relative standard error) of this estimate is much smaller—about one-quarter that of the two-week recall. (The exact reduction depends on the stability of individual visit patterns over time.)

We have tested for differences in bias by age, living arrangements (the latter would affect whether the respondent answered for himself or someone answered for him), and for all the other important explanatory variables in our regression models. Because there appeared to be no systematic pattern of bias differentials, we based our individual regressions on the twelve-month recall with no adjustments. For population estimates, we used population weights and the two-week recall, but never split into groups smaller than those aged 65 to 74 and those aged 75 and over.

Because the NHIS data base is very rich, we have a great deal of choice in picking variables to adjust our age differences. We developed the model on a random 20-percent sample of the data to see which variables appeared to be important. (We tried variables for region [South, Northwest, North Central, West]; location [central city, other SMSA (standard metropolitan statistical area), nonfarm non-SMSA, farm]; race; insurance status [not insured if 55 to 59, no Medicare, do not know if on Medicare]; family size; family income; family relationship [live alone, live with nonrelatives, live with spouse, live with other relatives]; a limitations-of-activity scale, a self-perceived health-status scale; education; interactions for family size and income; number of chronic conditions; and a variety of ways of fitting age [by polynomials interacted with sex and by age sex groups].) By rejecting those variables that do little to explain either hospital utilization or doctor visits, we reduced this list to the more manageable one shown in table B-2.

A final technical adjustment is to windsorize the hospital days and doctor visits to 30 (that is, those values greater than 30 were assigned the value of 30). This is done to prevent the few people with extremely large numbers of visits and days from dominating the results. Our main concern is the coefficients related to age. Table B-3 shows that, controlling for all the other variables, people aged 65 to 74 average 0.09 visit per year less than those aged 55 to 59, whereas people aged 75 and older average 0.2 visit less. Neither difference is statistically significant.

The results shown in the second panel of table B-3 indicate that old people are slightly more likely to go to the doctor at least once a year; but this difference is only marginally significant. The important determinants of the number of doctor visits are health related: each step on the self-reported health-status scale is associated with 1.2 doctor visits, and the number of restricted-activity days in the last two weeks is equally impor-

Table B-2
Statistics on Variables Used to Explain Utilization

Variable	Mean	Standard Deviation	Maximum
Self-perceived health status [a]	2.1	.9	4
Restricted-activity days in past two weeks	1.4	3.8	14
Limitation of activity scale [b]	3.1	1.2	4
Number of chronic conditions	.6	1.0	11
Family income scale [c]	7.2	2.7	11
Education scale [d]	4.3	1.3	7
Live in Southern region	0.32	NA	
Black or other race	0.09	NA	
Live alone or with nonrelative	0.23	NA	
Live with relatives but not spouse	0.14	NA	
Live outside of SMSA	0.35	NA	
Male, age 55-59	0.16	NA	
Male, age 65-74	0.19	NA	
Male, age 75 +	0.09	NA	
Female, age 65-74	0.24	NA	
Female, age 75 +	0.15	NA	

Notes: NA = dummy variables only.
Statistics for the ages we selected (55-59 and 65 +).
[a] (1) Poor; (2) fair; (3) good; (4) excellent.
[b] (1) Cannot perform usual activity; (2) limited in amount; (3) limited in outside activity; (4) not limited by chronic conditions.
[c] Scale runs from $1,000 or less = 1 to $25,000 + = 11
[d] Scale runs from none = 2 to college graduate = 7.

tant. Nonwhites have slightly more visits based on the yearly recall, but slightly fewer visits based on the two-week recall. The difference in annual and two-week recall suggests that nonwhites apparently forgot fewer visits or overestimated more than whites, although the standard error in two-week recall is large, approximately 10 percent. Rural people and Southerners have fewer visits. Chronic conditions have a substantial effect, particularly if they are serious enough to limit activity. Men have 0.8 fewer visits per year than women, on the average. In summary, these results show that, controlling for health status, old people go less often to the doctor, but that the difference is very small.

The hospital results are shown in table B-4. Even after controlling for health, those 65 yo 74 years old use about 0.5 day more per year than those 55 to 59 years old; and the older men use about 1.0 day per year more. Here,

Table B-3
Regression Results for Doctor Visits

Variable	Doctors Visits in Last Year (with 30 maximum)		Went to Doctor in Last Twelve Months?	
	Coefficient	t-Value	Coefficient	t-Value
Intercept	3.61	9	.695	25
Self-perceived health status	1.19	19	.042	10
Black or other race	.45	3	.012	1
Family income scale [a]	.05	4	.008	9
Restricted-activity days in past two weeks	.26	20	.006	7
Live outside SMSA	−.59	−6	−.018	−3
Live in Southern region	−.38	−4	−.006	−1
Live alone or with nonrelative	.43	4	.002	0
Live with relatives but not spouse	−.16	−1	.012	1
Education	.12	3	.025	9
Number of chronic conditions	.72	9	.021	4
Limitation-of-activity scale	−.69	−10	−.042	−9
Male	−.80	−8	−.071	−10
Age 65–74	−.09	−.8	.014	1.8
Age 75+	−.20	−1.5	.023	2.4
F-statistic	248		81	
R^2	.19		.07	
Degrees of freedom	14,655		14,655	

Source: Rand analysis of the National Health Interview Survey data (1976).
[a] Scale set to 0 if family size is larger than two persons.

the other health variables are still most important but do not seem to be as powerful in explaining utilization. This may be because they relate to continuing levels of health, whereas hospitalization is often due to an acute crisis that becomes more likely to occur as people age. For example, chronic conditions have almost no value in explaining hospital days. Nonwhites had fewer inpatient hospital days than whites.

This analysis showed that differences in sickness explain most of the difference in utilization between younger and older people, but it was unable to find any particularly underserved groups. It bears out the beneficial effects of Medicare that others have noted—increased hospital utilization by the elderly and a narrowing of differentials between rich and poor, black and white (Pettengill 1972; Wilson and White 1977).

On the basis of these findings, we have to generate two measures of utilization. The first is a simple projection based on the current utilization

Table B-4
Regression Results for Hospital Days

Variable	Hospital Days in Last Year (with 30 maximum)		Went to Hospital in Last Year?	
	Coefficient	t-Value	Coefficient	t-Value
Intercept	1.48	4	.118	5
Self-perceived health status	.61	11	.033	9
Black or other race	− .63	− 4	− .062	− 6
Restricted-activity days in past two weeks	.35	30	.020	26
Live outside of SMSA	.07	1	.022	4
Live in Southern region	− .19	− 2	− .003	0
Live alone or with nonrelative	.11	1	.009	1
Live with relatives but not spouse	.22	2	.007	1
Education	.15	4	.011	5
Number of chronic conditions	.01	0	.009	2
Limitation of activity scale	− .72	− 11	− .037	− 9
Female, age 65-74	.44	3.3	.012	1.3
Female, age 75 +	.48	3.0	.022	2.2
Male, age 55-59	.19	1.3	.004	0.4
Male, age 65-74	.51	3.6	.019	2.0
Male, age 75 +	1.04	5.9	.053	4.7
F-statistic	174		141	
R^2	.13		.11	
Degrees of freedom	16,810		16,810	

Source: Rand analysis of the National Health Interview Survey data (1976).

rates of the elderly. The second incorporates the age-specific utilization data and the differences in encounter time with age. The product of these two corrections is applied to the utilization rates to develop a measure termed "improved care." We note that this designation should not be confused with a direct manifestation of need for the reasons cited previously.

Demographic Predictions

Using census-bureau projections, we estimated the composition of the elderly population in 1977, 1990, 2010, and 2030. We could then apply the specific utilization rates for each age subgroup to estimate utilization for hospital and nonhospital care at each of the four dates. (There is no advantage in splitting groups into subgroups if there is no difference in utilization between the subgroups or if the proportion of the group in each subgroup does not change much over time. For this reason, we classify only by age groups because the sex ratio by age is expected to be fairly constant, and race and class differences in utilization are not substantial for the aged [Wilson and White 1977].)

Estimate of Current Utilization

Utilization can be estimated from the experience of recipients or providers. Because there are problems in each approach, we did it both ways. The NHIS asks about utilization for the noninstitutionalized (living) population. We supplemented this source with data collected by Medicare on utilization of decedents and estimates of nursing-home utilization. The estimates by provider were derived by combining the USC/DRME data on visits per doctor per week by type of physician with AMA data on the number of physicians of each type.

The estimates are obtained by dividing utilization into three parts. These parts consist of visits obtained by those alive and not institutionalized at the end of the year, those institutionalized in nursing homes at the end of the year (the NHIS includes those in hospitals), and those who died during the year. This partition is necessary because no single source gives the detail on conditions and utilization for all three groups. Luckily, the largest group by far, the living noninstitutionalized, is well covered by the NHIS. The other two groups each contain about 5 percent of the total aged population alive at some time during the year, and data on them are harder to obtain.

Level of utilization was calculated separately for nonhospital (outpatient and nursing-home visits) and acute hospital visits. Because we are not attempting to project surgical geriatric manpower, we excluded surgical visits from our estimates (for both supply and utilization).

We included psychiatry because of its importance in the care of the aged, but approached this estimate separately. Psychiatric practice is sufficiently different from either medical subspecialist or primary care in terms of productivity that data available on these two types of providers could not be safely extrapolated. Also, patterns of probable substitution for psychiatrists by other health care providers are entirely different.

Utilization Estimates Based on Recipient Reports

The first step was to find the factors to convert total short-stay hospital days to medical (nonsurgical) hospital visits, and total doctor visits to face-to-face medical-doctor visits. For hospitals, we estimated one medical visit per day in episodes without an operation, and one medical visit per episode with an operation if the episode is less than two weeks long. Longer episodes with an operation are assumed to generate one medical visit every other day on the average because of interservice transfers and extensive consultations. For people from nursing homes and those who died, we do not have details on the breakdown of hospital episodes into those with and without operations, so we assumed that the ratio of medical visits to hospital days is the same as for people in the NHIS. We have calculated this ratio to be 0.72 for persons aged 65 to 74 and 0.78 for those aged 75 and older.

We also needed to know the percentage of doctor visits to general practitioners or identified M.D. specialists other than surgical or psychiatric specialists. Table B-5 shows the responses to the question: "Is this doctor a general practitioner or a specialist?" Apparently, respondents were sometimes unaware that the doctor they were seeing was actually a surgeon. Psychiatric visits were also apparently underreported. Therefore, instead of these self-reported figures, we used the figure from the National Ambulatory Medical Care Survey (NAMCS) (Kovar 1977a) that people aged 65 and older saw a surgeon for 26 percent of their office visits and a psychiatrist for almost 1 percent. Thus the proportion of medical visits is really 73 percent, rather than the self-reported 80 percent. The assumed proportions are shown in table B-5, where the self-reports for each age are reduced by 0.730.8. A final adjustment consists of removing the 9.9 percent of "doctor visits" to the elderly that are actually telephone calls. Throughout, we have used only face-to-face encounters and have subtracted telephone calls from visits and from the available work time of physicians.

Nursing-home visits can be obtained simply from a survey of residents if we estimate one medical visit per month for those getting skilled care and one every two months for the rest. In the Survey of Institutionalized

Table B-5
Percentage of Nonhospital Doctor Visits That Are Medical and Psychiatric

Age Group	Self-Reported Visits		Provider-Reported Visits
	Medical [a]	Psychiatric	Medical[b]
65–74	78.0	.29	71.1
75 +	83.6	.16	76.2

Source: Our computations based on the National Health Interview Survey data (1976).

[a] Nonsurgical and nonpsychiatric. In this computation, osteopaths, "don't know doctor type," and "other specialties" were excluded from the denominator. In effect, these visits (9 percent) were split in the same way as the 91 percent that could be classified as medical, surgical, or psychiatric.

[b] Based on National Ambulatory Medical Care Survey data.

Patients, 65 percent of the institutionalized aged were getting monthly medical care (only 2.2 percent were getting psychiatric care monthly). This results in an assumption of (0.65 × 12) + (0.35 × 6) = 9.9 nursing-home visits per patient per year. Because 0.014 of patients 65 to 74 years old and 0.102 of those over 75 are in nursing homes (Hing and Zappolo 1978), we can multiply these numbers by 0.836, the percentage of medical-doctor visits for those 75 and older, and then by 9.9 to obtain the number of nursing-home visits per person shown in table B–6.

The doctor visits reported by the NHIS must be adjusted to include visits to decedents and to those who will enter nursing homes. The NHIS sample is picked at the beginning of the year, but interviews are conducted continuously throughout the year. Thus for data on the prevalence of conditions and doctor visits in the two weeks preceding the interview, they will miss one-half of the decedents and one-half of those who enter nursing homes to stay throughout the year. The Medicaid data presented later, and a 1961 report on disability and doctor visits of those who died in 1965 (Timmer and Kovar 1971), show that the rates are not more than three times as high. We assume that decedent doctor-visit rates are twice as high, that the rates for those who will enter a nursing home are 1.5 times as high, and that the visits are spread uniformly in the time prior to the time of institutionalization. Then the observed NHIS rates should be adjusted by the ratio $[1 + 0.5 (2D + 1.5N)]/[1 + 0.5 (D + N)]$, where D = the proportion of the age group who do not reside in nursing homes and who die, and N is the proportion who enter nursing homes to stay through the year. This ratio is 1.016 for those aged 65 to 74 and 1.042 for those over 75.

Finally, the entries in table B–6 come from multiplying

Age	× NHIS rate	× Factor	× Free-living fraction	× *Percentage Medical*	= Total
65–74	6.86	1.016	0.986	0.711	= 4.89
75+	6.78	1.042	0.898	0.762	= 4.83

The hospital estimates from the NHIS are low because of recall error and the large effect of decedents. Although we have elected to use the National Hospital Discharge Survey results (U.S. DHEW 1978c, table 102) for our calculations, there is some interest in how those who died during the calendar year and the institutionalized differ from the noninstitutionalized.

The major difference in utilization between those who died and those who did not is in the proportion that were hospitalized during the year. Piro's tabulations of Medicare reimbursements by age and survival status at the end of 1968 are summarized in table B–7 (Piro 1973). The difference in reimbursed expenses for physician services and other medical services was

Table B-6
Average Annual Medical Visits per Person, by Age and Locus

Age Group	Hospital Medical Visits [a]	Nursing-Home Medical Visits	Other Medical Visits	Total Nonhospital Face-to-Face Visits [b]
65–74	2.47	.12	4.89	4.51
75+	4.40	.84	4.83	5.11

[a] Based on nonfederal short-stay discharge data, adjusted for omitted federal short-stay days and for surgical days. The results from the National Health Interview Survey data (1976) on hospital visits (after correction for decedents) are 2.24 and 3.46, respectively.

[b] Total nonhospital medical visits, excluding telephone calls.

Table B-7
Hospital Utilization and Reimbursements Under Medicare for Persons Who Died in 1968 or Were Alive at the End of the Year

Hospital Utilization/Reimbursement	Age Group		
	Total	65–74	75+
Percentage hospital services utilized:			
Died	63	66	60
Alive at end of year	16	14	19
Inpatient hospital services reimbursed per person with episode:			
Died	$1160	$1250	$1100
Alive at end of year	$ 800	$ 840	$ 780
Average hospital reimbursement:			
Died	$ 731	$ 825	$ 660
Alive at end of year	$ 128	$ 109	$ 160
Ratio of dead/live hospital reimbursements	5.7	7.6	4.1

Source: P.A. Piro and T. Lutins, "Utilization and Reimbursements Under Medicare for Persons Who Died in 1967 and 1968," *Health Insurance Statistics Note HI-51,* Social Security Administration, October 17, 1973.

much smaller between decedents and the living aged. Decedents were about twice as likely (61 to 33) to have exceeded the deductible (then $50). The reimbursed expenses of those who died were $298 as opposed to $187 for those who did not. Because this reimbursement included physician and surgical fees at the hospital, the difference in out-of-hospital services is probably not too large.

Those who died had received 22.4 percent of all Medicaid reimbursements, but they were only 5.7 percent of enrollment that year. Interestingly, although total reimbursements for those alive at the end of the year rose with age, reimbursement for those dying fell with age (see table B-8). The Medicare statistics used by Piro count hospital expenses in the last calendar year for decedents, rather than in the preceding twelve months. Thus the correction for hospital use should be complete—the people interviewed by NHIS were all alive for the preceding twelve months, so that the ones missed because of death can be assumed to have had a higher proportion of hospital days compared with the living, just as in 1968. (Although expenses have increased since then, the share of large expenses has stayed fairly constant [Trapnell 1977].)

We were unable to find data on hospital utilization by nursing-home residents. An estimate based on the proportion of residents who entered homes from a hospital during the year and of those who went to the hospital temporarily without being formally discharged gave hospitalization rates for residents only slightly higher than rates for people of the same age who were free and living. For this reason, we assume that the NHIS hospitalization rates apply to all those persons alive at the end of the year.

All these assumptions on hospital medical visits lead to figures of total visits = NHIS visits × Factor for decedents = 3.13 visits for those 65 to 74 years old and 4.41 visits for those aged 75 and older. These numbers are substantially below the National Hospital Discharge Survey average of 1975-1976 (U.S. DHEW 1978b). Because of probable underreporting due to patients' foregetting in the NHIS, we will use the discharge data (collected at the hospitals) instead. These data give the average annual 1975-1976 number of nonfederal hospital days per noninstitutionalized person. Multiplying these data by the free-living fraction gives the days per person. Finally, because the federal short-stay hospitals were excluded, the totals were increased by 6.5 percent to include the 4.75 million Veterans Administration hospital days for those 65 and older and the estimated 2 million other such federal hospital days. The computations are as follows:

Age ×	Hospital days	Free-living ×	Federal ×	Medical visits per day	Hospital medical = visits per person
65–74	3.28	0.986	1.065	0.716	2.47
75+	5.86	0.898	1.065	0.784	4.40

Estimates of Utilization Based on Provider Reports

Estimates made on a provider-based method of the total utilization of primary-care physicians (PCP) and medical subspecialists (MSS) by patients aged 65 and older were performed as an independent verification of the estimates made by the consumer-based method.

Table B-8
Medicare Reimbursements in 1968, by Age and Survival Status

	Amount of Reimbursement	
Age Group	Alive at Year End	Died During Year
65–74	143	858
75–79	194	808
80–84	219	753
85 +	243	564
Total	167	764

The primary-care physician and medical subspecialist are synthetic physician types. The PCP is an aggregation of general practitioners, family practitioners, and internists. The medical subspecialist aggregates twelve medical specialties: allergy, cardiology, dermatology, endocrinology, gastroenterology, hematology, infectious disease, oncology, nephrology, neurology, pulmonology, and rheumatology.

The available data source for this material, the USC/DRME study, established the definitions of setting: hospital and nonhospital. The latter includes only inpatient encounters for nonfederal, acute-care hospitals. The nonhospital category includes physician office, clinics, nursing homes, and intermediate-care facilities. (Unfortunately, the Batelle study of the reliability and validity of the USC/DRME effort indicated that nursing-home visits were assigned by approximately half the physicians to the hospital category and by the other half to the nonhospital-visit category [Perrin 1978]. Thus any difference in characteristics of a visit attributable to its being in a nursing-home location would contaminate both hospital and nonhospital categories.)

In the USC/DRME study, physicians selected as a national stratified sample were asked to keep log diaries describing their use of time over a three-day period, either Monday through Wednesday or Thursday through Saturday. These data were then normalized to represent a typical, undifferentiated day in a six-day work week of the physician. The physician sample was selected to represent the physician population, thus permitting an extrapolation to national estimates. Table B-9 presents the nationally adjusted daily estimates of physician encounters with patients 65 years and older by physician type and setting.

To convert the daily number of encounters to annual encounters, we turned to data from the AMA. The *American Medical Association Annual Profile of Medical Practice, 1978,* reported the average number of work weeks per year at 47.2 (Gaffney 1979). This figure has remained stable since

1972. By using the USC/DRME's estimate of a typical work week composed of 6 days, we obtain a work year of 283.2 days. The USC/DRME estimate for conversion to annual utilization was 285, which was used here for purposes of consistency. The annual figures obtained by multiplying the figures for daily utilization in table B-9 by 285 are shown in table B-10.

Reconciliation of Provider-Based and Recipient-Based Estimates

The estimates of utilization derived from providers are considerably lower than those derived from the recipients. The main source of the difference is the physicians who fall between the cracks of the USC/DRME categories. These include federal physicians, interns, osteopaths, and those who either did not respond or did not indicate a specialty on the AMA questionnaires.

Table B-9
Daily Physician Encounters by Patients Aged 65 and Older, by Physician Type and Setting, 1976

Physician Type	Nonhospital Encounters	Hospital Encounters	Total Encounters
Internal medicine	92,636	92,816	185,452
General practice	132,740	49,592	182,332
Family practice	31,039	13,546	44,585
Cardiology	15,094	16,835	31,929
Dermatology	11,978	771	12,749
Pulmonology	2,929	4,359	7,288
Gastroenterology	2,632	4,129	6,761
Hematology	1,450	2,249	3,699
Medical oncology	851	1,161	2,012
Allergy	2,283	382	2,665
Rheumatology	1,494	852	2,346
Neurology	2,056	5,188	7,244
Endocrinology	680	849	1,529
Infectious disease	224	523	747
Nephrology	977	1,287	2,264
Primary care	256,415	155,954	412,369
Medical subspecialist	42,648	38,585	81,233
Total	299,063	194,539	493,602

Source: USC/DRME, *Practice Study Reports, Medical Activities and Manpower Project* (Los Angeles: USC School of Medicine, 1978).

Table B-10
Annual Physician Encounters by Patients Aged 65 and Older, by Physician Type and Setting, 1976

Type of Physician	Nonhospital Encounters	Hospital Encounters	Total Encounters
Primary-care physician	73,100,000	44,400,000	117,500,000
Medical subspecialist	12,200,000	11,000,000	23,200,000
Total	85,300,000	55,400,000	140,700,000

Table B-11
Estimates of Annual Medical Utilization for Patients Aged 65 and Older
(*Millions of visits*)

Type of Utilization	Nonhospital Visits	Hospital Visits
Provider-based, raw	85.3	55.4
Provider-based, adjusted	108.2	74.6
Recipient-based	111	75.8

Federal physicians supply 6.6 percent of the total patient care. Federal short-stay hospitals provided approximately 6.7 million days of care in 1977 to those over 65 years of age, which we estimate to include about 5 million medical visits. The federal physicians provide mainly hospital care, primarily through the VA, but may have provided another 1 percent of all nonhospital visits. Federal physicians make up about 0.75 percent of office-based patient-care physicians, and the VA provides about 185,000 outpatient visits per year to persons aged 65 and older. The AMA total patient-care category has another 9 percent more physicians than the population base used by USC/DRME (many of them are house staff). Osteopaths make up 4 percent of total doctors; they are included in NHIS estimates and should be included in ours. We do not include doctors who are temporarily abroad and those who are inactive, but we still must consider physicians "not classified" (those who did not respond to questionnaires), "unspecified" (those who did not indicate specialty), and those with "address unknown." These make up 11 percent of physicians. Assuming they fall into medical categories in the same proportion as respondents, they provide another 11 percent of care. The total of all of these adjustments is shown in table B-11. These estimates are reassuringly close for both hospital and nonhospital. We took the recipient figures of 111 and 75.8 million as our measure of current utilization.

Personnel Configurations

An important variable in the equation for estimating manpower demand is the partition of care among different types of physicians and nonphysicians. In chapter 3 we described four alternative levels of involvement of geriatricians in the care of the elderly, ranging from a minimal role (the status quo) to a very extensive role (in academic medical centers, in consultative practice, and in primary care). With each increment of geriatrician participation, the fraction of care delivered to the elderly by medical subspecialists and primary-care physicians must decline. For purposes of developing our boundary estimates, we have translated these qualitative descriptions into representative proportions of effort (table B-12). This quantification is admittedly arbitrary and is intended to provide a gross estimate of the distribution of workload for each assumed pattern of care.

Because team care has been widely advocated as a means of achieving more and better geriatric care, we have then proposed three possible patterns of shared workload between the geriatric specialist or the primary-care physician and geriatric nurse practitioners (GNPs), physician's assistants (PAs), or social workers (SWs) (table B-13). The minimum level corresponds roughly to the present situation. The medium and maximum levels of delegation are chosen to represent points on a spectrum without any specific practice model in mind. Experience to date with PAs and nurse practi-

Table B-12
Partition (Percentage) of Effort of Health-Care Personnel in the Care of the Elderly: Effect of Training Programs Aimed at Different Geriatrician Roles

Type of Training	Nonhospital Care [a]			Hospital Care		
	GS	MSS	PCP	GS	MSS	PCP
1. Status quo	1	14	85	1	19	80
2. Training geriatricians for academic positions only	—	—	—	—	—	—
3. Training geriatricians for academic positions and as consultants in practice	25	10	65	20	15	65
4. Training geriatricians for academic positions, as consultants and as primary-care physicians	40	10	50	30	15	55

Note: GS = geriatric specialist; MSS = medical subspecialist (cardiologist, gastroenterologist, and so on); PCP = primary-care physician (internist, family physician, general practitioner).
[a] Includes ambulatory care, nursing-home care, and common alternatives to nursing-home care.

Table B-13
**Partition (Percentage) of Effort of Health-Care Personnel in the Care of
the Elderly: Delegation of Physician Functions to Nonphysicians**

Level of Delegation	Nonhospital Care [a]			Hospital Care		
	MD [b]	PA/GNP [b]	SW [b]	MD	PA/GNP	SW
A. Minimal (status quo)	95	3	2	100	0	0
B. Moderate	65	25	10	90	10	0
C. Maximal	40	40	20	80	20	0

[a] Includes ambulatory care, outpatient, hospital, nursing-home care, and common alternatives
to nursing-home care.
[b] Only GS and PCP are assumed to delegate. MD refers only to nonsurgical physicians;
PA/GNP = physician assistant or geriatric nurse practitioner; SW = social worker.

tioners (NPs) suggests that no specific patterns of delegation of certain
types of patients over others is likely to occur. Except for the extent to
which the supervising physician sees the difficult cases of the PAs or NPs,
the practice profiles of the PAs and the NPs appear to be very similar to
that of the supervising physician. Medical subspecialists have not been
expected to delegate part of their work to these nonphysicians. To the extent
that the subspecialists may delegate, some of the physician model calls for
delegation of subspecialty work to the other physician categories.

Tables B-12 and B-13 can be combined to determine the number of
geriatric specialists, NPs, PAs, SWs, medical specialists, and primary-care
physicians who will be utilized under each of twelve possible combinations
of assumptions regarding the involvement of physicians and patterns of
delegation to nonphysicians. We will show how this is done by using case 3B
(table B-12, line 3 and table B-13, line B) as an example. Thus in the nonhospital locations, the 25 percent of care provided by geriatric specialists
and the 65 percent provided by primary-care physicians are further divided
to yield:

	GS	PA	SW	MSS
Calculation	0.25 × 65	0.25 × 25	0.25 × 10	0.10
Result (%)	16.25	6.25	2.5	10

	PCP	PA	SW
Calculation	0.65 × 65	0.65 × 25	0.65 × 10
Result (%)	42.25	16.25	6.5

By combining the NPs and PAs, and the SWs working with geriatric specialists and with primary-care physicians, we obtain the following partition of effort in case 3B:

	Percentage
GS	16.25
MSS	10
PCP	42.25
GNP/PA	22.5
SW	9.0

Similarly, in hospitals, the partition of effort in Case 3B is:

	Percentage
GS	18
MSS	15
PCP	58.5
GNP/PA	8.5
SW	0

The next step is to multiply these numbers by the number of medical visits required in each category in order to find the number of visits that could be handled by each category of worker. In 1990, for example, there will be 17.8 million persons aged 65 to 74 and 12.0 million aged 75 and older. If the current rates of utilization prevail, each person 65 to 74 years old will average 4.51 nonhospital visits and 2.47 hospital visits, and each person 75 and older will average 5.11 nonhospital visits and 4.40 hospital visits. Thus the total number of nonhospital visits expected in 1990 is $(17.8 \times 4.51) + (12.0 \times 5.11) = 141.6$ million visits; the total number of hospital visits expected in 1990 is $(17.8 \times 2.47) + (12.0 \times 4.40) = 96.8$ million. Finally, we multiply the fraction of effort for case 3B by the number of visits expected in 1990 to get the expected number of visits in each location handled by each type of provider. This yields 141.6 million $\times$ 0.1625 = 23 million nonhospital visits handled by geriatric specialists; $96.8 \times 0.18 = 17.5$ million hospital visits handled by geriatric specialists. The number of hospital and nonhospital visits expected to be handled by each type of provider in 1980 is shown below for case 3B:

	Millions of Visits	
	Nonhospital	*Hospital*
GS	23	17.5
MSS	14.2	14.5
PCP	59.8	56.6
GNP/PA	31.9	8.2
SW	12.7	0
Total	141.6	96.8

Productivity Estimates

From unpublished USC/DRME data, we were able to compute the average time per encounter with people aged 65 and over for primary-care physicians and to estimate it for medical specialists by using a weighted average of the twelve types of subspecialists who care for the largest number of elderly (cardiology, pulmonology, oncology, dermatology, gastroenterology, hematology, allergy, rheumatology, neurology, endocrinology, infectious disease, and nephrology). Because no comparable data are available for geriatric specialists, we estimated their productivity to be equal to that of the medical subspecialist. The productivity of GNP/PA and social worker is estimated on the basis of previous studies (Record and O'Bannon 1976; Golladay, Miller, and Smith 1973) at 60 percent of the corresponding physician's rate. We have not made any adjustment in physician needs to account for supervising time, however. These estimates are shown in table B-14.

The USC/DRME data also give information on face-to-face patient care per day. We put this on a per-week basis by multiplying the fraction of professional activity per week (excluding on call). Because we also know from AMA records that medical specialists and generalists average 47.4 weeks per year, we can multiply to get the total time spent in face-to-face care per year, as shown in table B-15.

By combining tables B-13 and B-14, we can estimate how many nonhospital visits a hypothetical provider who concentrated solely on nonhospital visits would provide in a year and how many hospital visits he would provide if he did nothing but hospital visits. (To be precise, we divide the total minutes per year by the minutes per encounter in that setting.) The results are shown in table B-15.

Finally, by dividing the number of visits per year in each location by the annual amount of care provided by each type of provider in that location,

Table B–14
Average Number of Minutes Spent per Patient per Encounter, by Type of Provider, Setting, and Age Group

Type of Provider	Minutes Spent with Nonhospital Patients[a]		Minutes Spent with Hospital Patients	
	Age 45–64	Age 65+	Age 45–64	Age 65+
Specialist	19.0	16.5	20.6	17.1
Primary-care physician	14.5	13.5	14.7	12.1
PA, GNP, SW[b]	24.2	22.5	24.5	20.2

Source: Our computations based on unpublished data provided by R.C. Mendenhall.
[a] Includes ambulatory, nursing home, clinic.
[b] Assumes productivity is 60 percent that of primary-care physician.

Table B–15
Amount of Patient Care Provided by Different Types of Providers

Type of Provider	Face-to-Face Care		Purely Nonhospital Visits	Purely Hospital Visits
	Hours per Week	Minutes per Year[a]		
Medical specialist	24.0	68,300	4140	3990
Primary-care physician	29.3	83,300	6170	6880
PA, GNP, SW	30	85,300	3790	4220
Psychiatrist	22.5	64,000	1600	2790

[a] Assumes 47.4 weeks per year.

we get the number of full-time equivalents (FTEs) needed for that location. Adding the two locations gives the total number of FTE providers of that type needed. This computation for full-time geriatricians for case 3B is as follows:

	Million Visits	Annual Productivity	FTEs
Hospital	23	4,140	5,556
Nonhospital	9.5	3,990	2,381
Total			7,937

This explanation has been tedious but, by using the appropriate formula, the computations can be done simply on a computer. One final wrinkle in our results should be mentioned. In cases 3 and 4 (table B-12), we assume that an academic program is in place employing 900 trained geriatricians. Because these are assumed to devote 25 percent of their time to patient care, the other 75 percent (or 675 FTEs) is missing. Thus, all the estimates in cases 3 and 4 have had 675 added to them to reflect the numbers required for academia.

Having developed estimates of manpower needed to match current utilization and productivity, we then sought methods to estimate manpower needed for care at a more nearly optimal level. As discussed earlier, there is no ideal way to do this. The data on doctor-patient encounters (table B-14) provided a clue to one component of optimization. Note that average contact was 1 to 3 minutes briefer for patients 65 years and older than for middle-aged patients. This difference was consistent throughout nine different specialties, for hospital and nonhospital encounters, for several degrees of care complexity and severity, and for most types of encounters. Assuming that the longer times spent on patients aged 45 to 64 represent better care, we introduced the ratio of encounter times for the two age groups as a multiplier to derive an estimate for more optimal care.

In addition, the elderly underutilize services to a slight degree. Adjusted for their levels of illness, old people have somewhat fewer nonhospital visits. If the rates of nonhospital physician visits increase to those for persons aged 55 to 59 (adjusted for illness), they become 4.91 for those under age 75 and 5.97 for those 75 years and older. Because the hospital-visit rates are already greater, they remain the same for our estimate of improved care.

We combined the correction ratio for encounter time with that for underutilization to provide an estimate of manpower needs for more optimal care. This estimate yields two multipliers: 1.26 for the total population aged 65 and older, and 1.28 if only those aged 75 and older are addressed.

Appendix C:
Objectives of a Geriatric
Fellowship

Each of the behavioral objectives listed in this appendix should be read with "The fellow will be able to . . ." preceding each statement:

I. Clinical knowledge
  A. Physiology and pathophysiology
    1. Delineate the following theories and mechanisms of aging:
       a. Free radical
       b. Genetic
       c. Immunological
       d. Endocrine
       e. Collagen cross-linking
    2. Distinguish "normal" aging from pathology
       a. Given a clinical scenario, distinguish pathology from "normal" aging
       b. Describe the changes in each organ system expected in a modal individual from ages 50 to 90
       c. Distinguish functional from chronological age
    3. Describe the pathophysiology of the following diseases:
       a. Dementia
       b. Cerebrovascular disease
       c. Arteriosclerotic heart disease
       d. Congestive heart failure
       e. Arrhythmias
       f. Anemia
       g. Chronic obstructive pulmonary disease
       h. Respiratory failure, acute and chronic
       i. Diabetes mellitus
       j. Thyroid disease
       k. Hypertension
       l. Chronic renal insufficiency
       m. Degenerative joint disease
       n. Rheumatoid arthritis, gout and pseudogout, polymyaglia rheumatica, and temporal arteritis
       o. Osteoporosis
       p. Malignancy
       q. Prostatic disease
       r. Glaucoma and cataract
       s. Decreased hearing and deafness
       t. Geriatric gynecology

       u. Depression and anxiety
       v. Geriatric dermatology
      w. Alcoholism and drug abuse
       x. Sensory deprivation
       y. Functional disorders
       z. Infections in the elderly
      aa. Peripheral vascular disease
      bb. Geriatric orthopedics
    4. Describe the effect of dysfunction in one organ on the function of other organs

B. Clinical pharmacology
    1. Describe changes associated with aging in drug absorption, transport, metabolism, and excretion
    2. Describe specific drug groups and related organs of metabolism
    3. Describe common side effects of certain categories of drugs in the elderly
    4. Describe factors associated with compliance in the elderly
    5. Describe treatment options other than drugs

C. Psychosocial
    1. Describe changes in cognitive function found in modal group of aging individuals
    2. Describe the norms of sexual behavior in patients of various ages beyond 60
    3. Describe the major changes in life-style and social role often encountered in the elderly; suggest actions that may be useful in ameliorating each
    4. Describe the stages of bereavement and the Kubler-Ross model for the individual's manner of coping with death and dying
    5. Describe the various ways in which society may show a negative bias toward the elderly
    6. List the social characteristics that distinguish elderly individuals at greatest risk of illness and institutionalization
    7. Discuss the health-belief model and its use in caring for the elderly
    8. Describe the problems faced by the elderly in the following areas: housing, transportation, obtaining medical care, economics, social needs, and general needs for services (see II.H)

D. Preventive medicine: Describe a program to detect asymptomatic disease; justify choice of tests in terms of efficacy and frequency of use

II. Clinical skills
   A. Obtain and record an accurate medical history in the elderly so as
      to exhibit the following behaviors:
      1. Recognize the reason for the visit
      2. Obtain a complete description of all pertinent problems,
         exploring relevant leads
      3. Assess reliability of patient's history and consult significant
         other if necessary
      4. Obtain relevant past medical history, including diet and drug
         history
      5. Perform a detailed review of systems, accurately assessing
         multiple pathology
      6. Obtain a psychosocial history to include an assessment of
         finance, housing, transportation, support from social services,
         family support, nature of personal relationships, and degree of
         isolation, as well as evaluation of personality, motivation,
         mobility, daily activities, interests and hobbies, sexual prac-
         tices; specific questions asked related to depression, sleep prob-
         lems, appetite, weight loss, self-care
      7. Determine the functional capacity of the patient in regard to
         physical and psychosocial disabilities
   B. Demonstrate communication and interpersonal skills by exhibiting
      the following behaviors during a medical interview:
      1. Introduce self and put patient at ease
      2. Allow patient to verbalize, listen attentively, and use open-
         ended questions
      3. Provide an unhurried approach, conveying a feeling of warmth
         and concern
      4. Minimize medical jargon, discuss diagnostic and therapeutic
         plans with patient
      5. Provide physical contact when necessary and frequently reas-
         sure and support
      6. Address the relevant emotional factors of illness by demon-
         strating awareness of interpersonal issues
      7. Provide the patient with information in a clear, concise manner
         and check the patient's understanding of this information
      8. Demonstrate techniques for encouraging elderly patients to
         communicate their feelings and the problems they are encoun-
         tering
   C. Perform and record a complete physical examination in the elderly
      with specific regard to the following systems:

System	*Special Emphasis*
1. General	Observe state of nutrition, evidence of neglect or trauma, posture, spontaneity, mobility, careful check of blood pressure, rate and rhythm of pulse
2. Skin	Observe for xerosis, excoriations, ischemic changes, decubiti, skin tumors
3. Eyes	Check visual acuity and measurement of pressure, confrontation test, lens for cataracts
4. ENT	Check hearing acuity, bone and air conduction; check dentition, oral lesions
5. Respiratory	Check chest deformity, force of cough, presence and type of sputum, restriction of chest movement
6. Cardiovascular	Characterization of murmurs; quantification of pulses, listen for bruits
7. Gastrointestinal (GI)	Palpate for abdominal pulsations; rectal for masses, fecal impaction
8. Genitourinary (GU)	Palpate and percuss for bladder, characterize prostate and note rectal sphincter tone; perform pelvic examination
9. Extremities	Asses joint deformities, mobility, range of motion (ROM), muscle strength, tone, and mass; observe lower extremities for edema, varicosities and tenderness in legs, examine feet for callouses, ulceration, neglect
10. Back	Observe for deformity, mobility, vertebral tenderness
11. Neurologic	Speech assessment, tremor, gait, frontal lobe release signs; mental status examination, including orientation, memory, intellectual function, behavior, and mood

D. Describe the differential diagnosis and appropriate evaluation steps for common symptom complexes in the elderly, for example:

1. Anorexia
2. Insomnia
3. Pain syndromes
4. Fatigue
5. Dizziness
6. Weight loss
7. Disorientation
8. Apathy
9. Fear/suspicion
10. Anxiety

E. Devise and conduct a diagnostic workup and carry out a therapeutic plan for the following medical and psychological disorders in the elderly:

1. Dementia
2. Seizure disorders
3. Cerebrovascular disease
4. Parkinsonism
5. Peripheral neuropathy
6. Arteriosclerotic heart disease
7. Cardiomyopathy
8. Congestive heart failure
9. Valvular disease
10. Arrhythmias
11. Anemia
12. Chronic obstructive pulmonary disease
13. Respiratory failure, acute and chronic
14. Diabetes mellitus
15. Thyroid disease
16. Hypertension
17. Pneumonia, bronchitis
18. Urinary tract infection
19. Functional bowel disease
20. Diverticulitis
21. Peptic ulcer disease
22. Peripheral vascular disease
23. Venous insufficiency and thrombosis, thrombophlebitis
24. Chronic renal insufficiency
25. Degenerative joint disease
26. Rheumatoid arthritis, gout and pseudogout, polymyalgia rheumatica, and temporal arteritis
27. Osteoporosis
28. Malignancy
29. Prostatic disease
30. Cataract and glaucoma

31. Decreased hearing and deafness
32. Geriatric gynecology
33. Depression
34. Geriatric dermatology
35. Sensory deprivation
36. Geriatric orthopedics
37. Alcoholism and drug abuse
38. Evaluation of elderly patients for surgery

F. Maintain an organized, legible, problem-oriented medical record including a problem list, assessment progress notes, and a complete drug profile (both prescribed and over-the-counter medication)

G. Maintain medical records to reflect timely awareness of nursing notes, referrals, and diagnostic information

H. Counsel and/or refer elderly patients to the appropriate allied health personnel and resources in regard to the following areas:
   1. Housing, transportation, meals
   2. Family, marriage, sex, isolation
   3. Financial assistance, senior-citizen organizations
   4. Public-health screening and preventive medicine
   5. Physical medicine and rehabilitation
   6. Self-help groups; social and hobby clubs
   7. Options for health care—institutions, home care, after care, and so on
   8. Death and dying
   9. Retirement, life adjustment, and stresses
   10. Ethnic and religious issues
   11. Employment and occupational therapy
   12. Dietetics
   13. Dentistry
   14. Podiatry
   15. Alcoholism

I. Demonstrate evidence of continuous monitoring of patient compliance (for example, patient inquiry, pill count, and drug levels)

J. In devising a therapeutic plan, demonstrate appreciation of the implications of medical care

K. Given a clinical problem, outline a rehabilitation plan, including the description of each participant's role

L. Given a patient with a new diagnosis and existing drug regimen (including both prescribed and over-the-counter drugs), describe and defend a new drug regimen, including choice of drug, dosage, interval, and route

III. Clinical attitudes
   A. Identify and eliminate fellow's own biases and misconceptions about the elderly
   B. Recognize and improve on deficiencies in interpersonal awareness and empathy
   C. Identify and deal with fellow's own fear of aging, death, and dying
   D. Develop a sense of responsibility in caring for the elderly and implement a follow-up system to assess the outcomes of patient care
   E. Structure priorities, develop interest and gratification in providing health care for the aged
   F. Recognize the role of the physician as a member of a health-care team, collaborating with allied health personnel, and using numerous resources to optimize health care

IV. Teaching knowledge
   A. Describe the basic principles of learning
   B Describe the development of an educational program in geriatrics
   C. Discuss teaching methods available
   D. Relate the principles of program evaluation
   E. Discuss educational activity in geriatrics on a local and national level

V. Teaching skills
   A. Present relevant material at conferences and rounds (in group or individual sessions) in an organized, understandable fashion that stimulates interest and thought in topics discussed
   B. Guide, counsel, and interact with students to promote the learning process
   C. Implement and organize an educational program on a geriatric topic, including specifying learning objectives, assessing effectiveness of the programs, and devising a plant to improve learning
   D. Act as a clinical role model, demonstrating positive attitudes toward patient care and skills in interviewing and physical examinations as previously outlined

VI. Teaching attitudes
   A. Foster the fellow's own interest and enthusiasm for teaching
   B. Develop a sensitivity to the feelings of others, their problems and concerns
   C. Recognize and modify the fellow's own tendency toward authoritarian teaching and develop respect for the opinions of others
   D. Recognize the important role of the health educator in forming habits of medical practice and affecting health-care policy

VII. Scholarship
   A. Evaluate care being given in terms of process and outcomes
   B. Evaluate report of an assessment performed by others (external review, paper)
   C. Design and conduct a simple study of some aspect of geriatric care or of disease
   D. Write an organized, critical, thorough review of a clinically related topic on the aged
VIII. Administrative
   A. Prepare a budget
   B. Write a job description for each major professional on the geriatric health-care team
   C. Describe the forces that affect patient care in different institutions: nursing home, old-age home, acute hospital, day-care center
   D. Participate as a member of a health-care team
   E. Participate as a leader of a health-care team
   F. Given a case scenario, outline an investigation and treatment plan that includes the roles of appropriate professionals
   G. Describe a clinical-record system for monitoring case and patient progress
   H. Demonstrate effective communication skills with health-care workers
   I. Outline the eligibility criteria and benefits provided by Medicare and Medicaid (Medi-Cal)
   J. Carry out a geriatric consultation and prepare a report
   K. Request a consultation and make a referral, providing all pertinent data

Appendix D:
Objectives for Internal-Medicine Residents and Medical Students

The outline should be read with "The resident will be able to . . ." preceding each objective

I. Clinical knowledge
  A. Physiology and pathophysiology
     *1. Briefly delineate the following theories and mechanisms of aging:
        a. Free radical
        b. Genetic
        c. Immunological
        d. Endocrine
        e. Collagen cross-linking
      2. Distinguish "normal aging" from pathology
        *a. Given a clinical scenario, distinguish pathology from "normal" aging
         b. Describe the changes in each organ system expected in a modal individual from ages 50 to 90
         c. Distinguish functional from chronological age
     *3. Describe the pathophysiology of the following diseases:
        a. Dementia
        b. Cerebrovascular disease
        c. Chronic renal insufficiency
        d. Degenerative joint disease
        e. Polymyalgia rheumatica
        f. Osteoporosis
        g. Malignancy
        h. Prostatis disease
        i. Cataract and glaucoma
        j. Decreased hearing and deafness
        k. Geriatric gynecology
        l. Depression and anxiety
        m. Geriatric dermatology
        n. Sensory deprivation
        o. Alcoholism and drug abuse.
        p. Functional disorders

Those items preceded by an asterisk are objectives for medical students.

        q. Infections in the elderly

        r. Peripheral vascular disease

        s. Geriatric orthopedics

    4. Describe the effect of dysfunction in one organ on the function of other ograns

  B. Clinical pharmacology

    *1. Describe changes associated with aging in drug absorption, transport, metabolism, and excretion

    *2. Describe specific drug groups and related organs of metabolism

    3. Given a patient with a new diagnosis and existing drug regimen (including prescribed and over-the-counter drugs), describe and defend a new drug regimen in terms of choice of drug, dosage, interval, and route

    4. Describe common side effects of certain categories of drugs in the elderly

    *5. Describe factors associated with compliance in the elderly

    6. Describe treatment options other than drug

*C. Psychosocial

    1. Describe changes in cognitive function found in a modal group of aging individuals

    2. Describe the norms of sexual behavior in patients of various ages beyond 60

    3. Describe the major changes in life-style and social role often encountered in the elderly; suggest actions that may be useful in ameliorating each

    4. Describe the stages of bereavement and the Kubler-Ross model for the individual's manner of coping with death and dying

    5. Describe the various ways in which society may show a negative bias toward the elderly

    6. List the social characteristics that distinguish elderly individuals at greatest risk of illness and institutionalization

    7. Discuss the health-belief model and its use in caring for the elderly

    8. Describe the problems faced by the elderly in the following areas: housing, transportation, obtaining medical services, economics, social needs, general needs for services

    9. Contrast the demographic characteristics of institutionalized elderly populations

    10. Describe the effects of institutionalization on the elderly patient and distinguish the effects of different types of institutions

II. Clinical skills: Counsel and/or refer elderly patients to the appropriate
    allied health personnel and resources in regard to the following areas:
    A. Housing, transportation, meals
    B. Family, marriage, sex, isolation
    C. Financial assistance, senior-citizen organizations
    D. Public-health screening and preventive medicine
    E. Physical medicine and rehabilitation
    F. Self-help groups; social and hobby clubs
    G. Options for health care—institutions, home care, after care, and
       so on
    H. Death and dying
    I. Retirement, life adjustment, and stresses
    J. Ethnic and religious issues
    K. Employment and occupational therapy
    L. Dietetics
    M. Dentistry
    N. Podiatry
    O. Alcoholism

Bibliography

Aiken, L.H.; Lewis, C.E.; Craig, J.; Mendenhall, R.C.; Blendon, R.J.; and Rogers, D.E. "The Contribution of Specialists to the Delivery of Primary Care." *New England Journal of Medicine* 300(1979):363–370.

Akpom, C.A., and Meyer, S. "A Survey of Geriatric Education in the United States Medical Schools." *Journal of Medical Education* 53 (1978):66–68.

Anderson, W.F. *Practical Management of the Elderly.* Oxford: Blackwell Scientific Publications, 1971.

Binstock, R.H. "Federal Policy Toward the Aging." *National Journal,* November 11, 1978, pp. 1838–1845.

Binstock, R.H., and Shanas, E., eds. *Handbook of Aging and the Social Sciences.* New York, Van Nostrand Reinhold, 1976.

Birren, J.E., and Schaie, K.W., eds. *Handbook of the Psychology of Aging.* New York: Van Nostrand Reinhold, 1977.

Birren, J.E., and Sloane, R.B. *Manpower and Training Needs in Mental Health and Illness of the Aging.* Los Angeles: Ethel Percy Andrus Gerontology Center, 1977.

Bloom, M. "Evaluation Instruments: Tests and Measurements in Long-Term Care," in *Long-Term Care: Handbook for Researchers, Planners and Providers,* ed. S. Sherwood, pp. 573–638. New York: Spectrum Publications, 1975.

Brocklehurst, J.C.; Carthy, M.H.; Leeming, J.T.; and Robinson, J.M. "Medical Screening of Old People Accepted for Residential Care." *Lancet* (1978):141–143.

Bunker, J.P. "Surgical Manpower: A Comparison of Operations and Surgeons in the United States and in England and Wales." *New England Journal of Medicine* 282(1970):135–140.

Butler, R. *Why Survive: Being Old in America.* New York: Harper & Row, 1975.

———. "The Economics of Aging: We Are Asking the Wrong Questions." *National Journal,* November 4, 1978, pp. 1792–1797.

Califano, J.A. "U.S. Policy for the Aging." *National Journal,* September 30, 1978, pp. 1575–1581.

Chisholm, R.N. "The History of Family Practice." in *Family Medicine: Principles and Practice,* ed. R.B. Taylor, pp. 7–12. New York: Springer-Verlag, 1978.

Clark, R.; Kreps, J.; and Spengler, J. "Economics of Aging: A Survey." *Journal of Economic Literature* 16(1978):919–962.

Coccaro, E.F. *Clinical Geriatrics Training Sites Directory.* Chantilly, Va.: American Medical Student Association, 1979.

Dans, P.E., and Kerr, M.R. "Gerontology and Geriatrics in Medical Education." *New England Journal of Medicine* 300(1979):228-232.

Darley, W. "Family Physicians of the Future: Fact or Fiction." *Journal of Medical Education* 36(1961):142-149.

Duke University Center for the Study of Aging and Human Development. *Multidimensional Functional Assessment: The OARS Methodology.* Durham, N.C.: Duke University, 1978.

Eddy, D.M. "Screening for Cancer: Theory, Analysis, and Design," Mimeographed 1979.

Eisdorfer, C "The Future of Aging and the Training of Health Care Professionals." Joseph T. Freeman Lecture delivered at the Gerontological Society Annual Meeting, Washington, D.C., 1979.

Engel, G.L. "The Need for a New Medical Model: A Challenge for Biomedicine." *Science* 196(1977):129-136.

Federal Council on Aging. *Public Policy and the Frail Elderly.* DHEW Publication no. (OHDS) 79-20959. Washington, D.C.: U.S. Government Printing Office, 1978.

Finch, C.E., and Hayflick, L., eds. *Handbook of the Biology of Aging.* New York: Van Nostrand Reinhold, 1977.

Freeman, J.T. "A Survey of Geriatric Education: Catalogues of United States Medical Schools." *Journal of the American Geriatrics Society* 19(1971):746-762.

Fry, J. *Medicine in Three Societies—A Comparison of Medical Care in the USSR, USA, and UK.* New York: American Elsevier Publishing Company, 1970.

Gaffney, J.C., ed. *Profile of Medical Practice, 1978.* Chicago: AMA Center for Health Services Research and Development, 1979.

George, L.K. "The Happiness Syndrome: Methodological and Substantive Issues in the Study of Social Psychological Well-Being in Adulthood." *The Gerontologist* 19(1979):210-216.

Gibson, R.M., and Fisher, C.R. "Age Differences in Health Care Spending, Fiscal Year 1977." *Social Security Bulletin* 42(1979):3-16.

Golladay, F.L.; Miller, M.; Smith, K.R. "Allied Health Manpower Strategies: Estimates of the Potential Gains from Efficient Task Delegation." *Medical Care* 11(1973):457-469.

Goodman, L.J. *Physician Distribution and Medical Licensure in the United States, 1977.* Chicago: American Medical Association, 1979.

Goran, M.; Crystal, R.; Ford, L.; and Tebbutt, J. "PSRO Review of LTC Utilization and Quality." *Medical Care* 14(1976):94-98.

Graduate Medical Education National Advisory Committee (GMENAC). *Interim Report to the Secretary.* DHEW Publication no. (HRA) 79-633. Washington, D.C.: U.S. Government Printing Office, 1979.

Graney, M.J., and Graney, E.E. "Scaling Adjustment in Older People." *International Journal on Aging and Human Development* 4(1973):351-359.

Guide to Family Practice Residency Programs. American Academy of Family Physicians and American Medical Student Association, 1979.

Gunter, L.M., and Estes, C.A. *Education for Gerontic Nursing.* New York: Springer Publishing Company, 1979.

Gutkin, C.; Morris, J.N.; Sherwood, S.; and Stone, R. "A Mathematical Function to Predict Potential of Transfer to a Community Care Home for Level II Nursing Home Patients in Vermont." Draft paper, January 30, 1979.

Hing, E., and Zappolo, A. "A Comparison of Nursing Home Residents and Discharges from the 1977 National Nursing Home Survey: United States." DHEW Publication no. (PHS) 78-1250. Advance data from *Vital and Health Statistics of the National Center for Health Statistics,* no. 29, May 17, 1978, pp. 1-8.

Hudson, R.B. "Political and Budgetary Consequences of an Aging Population." *National Journal,* October 21, 1978, pp. 1699-1705.

Hughes, E.F.; Lewit, E.M.; Watkins, R.N.; and Handschin, R. "Utilization of Surgical Manpower in a Prepaid Group Practice." *New England Journal of Medicine* 291(1974):759-761.

Institute of Medicine (IOM). *Aging and Medical Education.* Washington, D.C.: National Academy of Sciences, 1978.

———. *A Survey of US Medical School Programs in Geriatrics and Gerontology.* Washington, D.C.: National Academy of Sciences, 1979.

Isaacs, B.; Livingstone, M.; and Neville, Y. *Survival of the Unfittest: A Study of Geriatric Patients in Glasgow.* London: Routledge & Kegan Paul, 1972.

Jick, H. "The Discovery of Drug-Induced Illness." *New England Journal of Medicine* 296(1977):481-485.

Jones, E.; McNitt, B.; McKnight, E. *Patient Classification for Long-term Care: User's Manual.* DHEW Publication no. (HRA) 75-3107. Washington, D.C.: U.S. Government Printing Office, 1974.

Kane, R.A. *Consequential Decisions of Older Persons: A Framework for Study.* P-6233. Santa Monica, Calif.: Rand Corporation, 1978.

Kane, R.A.; Kane, R.L.; Kleffel, D.; Brook, R.; Eby, C.; Goldberg, G.; Rubenstein, L.; and Van Ryzin, J. *The PSRO and the Nursing Home.* R-2459/1-HCFA. Santa Monica, Calif.: Rand Corporation, 1979.

Kane, R.L., and Kane, R.A. *Assessing the Elderly: A Practical Guide to Measurement.* Lexington, Mass.: Lexington Books, D.C. Heath, 1981.

Kane, R.L., and Kane, R.A. "Alternatives to Institutional Care of the Elderly: Beyond the Dichotomy." *The Gerontologist* 20(1980):249-259.

Kane, R.L.; Dean, M.; and Solomon, M. "An Evaluation of Rural Health Care Research." *Evaluation Quarterly* 3(1979):139-189.

Kane, R.L.; Hammer, D.; and Byrnes, N. "Getting Care to Nursing Home Patients: A Problem and a Proposal." *Medical Care* 15(1977):174-180.

Kane, R.L.; Jorgensen, L.A.; Teteberg, B; and Kuwahara, J. "Is Good

Nursing-Home Care Feasible?" *Journal of the American Medical Association* 235 (1976a):516-519.

Kane, R.L.; Woolley, F.R.; Hughes, C.C.; Schmidt, L.J.; and Ryssman, A.L. "Communication Patterns of Doctors and their Assistants." *Medical Care* 14 (1976b):348-356.

Katz, S.; Hedrick, S.; and Henderson, N. "The Measurement of Long-Term Care Needs and Impact." *Health and Medical Care Services Review* 2(1979):2-21.

Kent, D.; Kastenbaum, R.; and Sherwood, S., eds. *Research Planning and Action for the Elderly.* New York: Behavioral Publications, 1972.

Klarman, H.E. "Approaches to Moderating the Increases in Medical Care Costs." *Medical Care* 7(1969):177-179.

Kovar, M.G. "Elderly People: The Population 65 Years and Over." in *Health, United States, 1976-1977.* DHEW Publication no. (HRA) 77-1232. Washington, D.C.: U.S. Government Printing Office, 1977a.

———. "Health of the Elderly and the Use of Health Services." *Public Health Reports* 92(1977b):9-19.

Larson, R. "Thirty Years of Research on the Subjective Well-Being of Older Americans." *Journal of Gerontology* 33(1978):109-125.

Libow, L.S. "Testimony at Joint Hearing Before the Subcommittee on Health and Long-term Care and the Subcommittee on Human Services of the Select Committee on Aging, House of Representatives, May 17, 1978." Committee Publication no. 95-151. Washington, D.C.: U.S. Government Printing Office, 1978.

Maddox, G.L., and Dellinger, D.C. "Assessment of Functional Status in a Program Evaluation and Resource Allocation Model." *Annals of the American Academy of Political and Social Science* 438(1978):59-70.

Mager, R.F. *Preparing Instructional Objectives.* Palo Alto, Calif.: Fearon Publishers, 1962.

Mark, R.G.; Willemain, T.R.; Malcolm, T.; Master, R.J.; and Clarkson, T. *Final Report of the Nursing Home Telemedicine Project,* vol. 1. Washington, D.C.: National Science Foundation, 1976.

McNeil, B.; Weichselbaum, R.; and Pauker, S. "Fallacy of Five-Year Survival in Lung Cancer." *New England Journal of Medicine* 299(1978): 1397-1401.

Mendenhall, R.C.; Girard, R.A.; and Abrahamson, S. "A National Study of Medical and Surgical Specialties. I: Background, Purpose, and Methodology." *Journal of the American Medical Association* 240 (1978):848-852.

Mendenhall, R.C.; Lloyd, J.S.; Repicky, P.A.; Monson, J.R.; Girard, R.A.; and Abrahamson, S. "A National Study of Medical and Surgical Specialties, II: Description of the Survey Instruments." *Journal of the American Medical Association* 240(1978):1160-1168.

Millis, J.S. *The Graduate Education of Physicians: The Report of the Citizens' Commission on Graduate Medical Education.* Chicago: American Medical Association, 1966.

Moscovice, I. "The Influence of Training Level and Practice Setting on Patterns of Primary Health Care Provided by Nursing Personnel." *Journal of Community Health* 4(1978):4-14.

National Commission on Community Health Services. *Health Is a Community Affair.* Cambridge, Mass.: Harvard University Press, 1966.

National Institute on Aging (NIA). *Our Future Selves: A Research Plan Toward Understanding Aging.* Publication no. (NIH) 78-1444. Washington, D.C.: U.S. Government Printing Office, 1978.

———. *Special Report on Aging, 1979.* Publication no. 79-1907. Washington, D.C.: U.S. Government Printing Office, 1979.

Olsen, D.M.; Kane, R.L.; and Kasteler, J. "Medical Care as a Commodity: An Exploration of the Shopping Behavior of Patients." *Journal of Community Health* 2(1976):85-91.

Palmore, E. ed. *Normal Aging Reports from the Duke Longitudinal Study, 1955-1969.* Durham, N.C.: Duke University Press, 1970.

———. *Normal Aging II: Reports from the Duke Longitudinal Studies, 1970-1973.* Durham, N.C.: Duke University Press, 1974.

Perrin, E.B.; Harkins, E.B.; and Marini, M.M. *Evaluation of the Reliability and Validity of Data Collected in the USC Medical Activities and Manpower Projects.* Seattle, Wash.: Health and Population Study Center, Battelle Human Affairs Research Centers, 1978.

Pettingill, J.H. "Trends in Hospital Use by the Aged." *Social Security Bulletin* 35(1972):3-15.

Pfeiffer, E. "The Need for Faculty Development in Geriatric Medicine." *Journal of the American Geriatrics Society* 25(1977):490-491.

Piro, P.A., and Lutins, T. "Utilization and Reimbursements Under Medicare for Persons Who Died in 1967 and 1968." *Health Insurance Statistics Note HI-51,* Social Security Administration, October 17, 1973.

Pisacano, N.J. "The American Board of Family Practice." in *Family Medicine: Principles and Practice,* ed. R.B. Taylor. New York: Springer-Verlag, 1978.

Pollak, W. *Expanding Health Benefits for the Elderly,* vol. 1: *Long-Term Care.* Washington, D.C.: Urban Institute, 1979.

Raskin, A., and Jarvik, L.F. *Psychiatric Symptoms and Cognitive Loss in the Elderly.* Washington, D.C.: Hemisphere Publishing Corporation, 1979.

Record, J.C., and O'Bannon, J.E. *Cost Effectiveness of Physicians' Assistants, Final Report.* Health Manpower Education Initiative Award, 1976.

Reichel, W. "Final Recommendations of the American Geriatrics Society

Conference on Geriatric Education, March 4–5, 1977." *Journal of the American Geriatrics Society* 25(1977):510–512.

Robbins, A.S.; S. Vivell; R.L. Kane; I. Abrass; A. Fink; J. Kosecoff; and J.C. Beck. *Geriatric Medicine: An Education Resource Guide.* Cambridge, Mass.: Ballinger, 1981.

Roemer, M.I. "Bed Supply and Hospital Utilization: A Natural Experiment." *Hospitals* 35(1960):36–42.

Rogers, D.E. "On Preparing Academic Health Centers for the Very Different 1980s." *Journal of Medical Education* 55(1980):1–12.

Sadler, A.M.; Sadler, B.L.; and Bliss, A.A. *The Physician's Assistant Today and Tomorrow,* 2d ed. Cambridge, Mass.: Ballinger Publishing Company, 1975.

Salzman, C.; Shader, R.T.; Kochansky, G.E.; and Cronin, D.M. "Rating Scales for Psychotropic Drug Research with Geriatric Patients. I: Behavior Ratings." *Journal of the American Geriatrics Society* 20 (1972):209–214.

Scheele, G.A., and Kitzes, G. "Analysis of Academic Training Programs in Gastroenterology for the Ten-Year Period 1957–1967." *Gastroenterology* 57(1969):203–224.

Scheffler, R.M.; Yoder, S.G.; Weisfeld, N.; and Ruby, G. "Physicians and New Health Practitioners: Issues for the 1980's." *Inquiry* 16(1979): 195–229.

Schwartz, W.; Newhouse, J.; Bennett, B.; and Williams, A. "The Changing Geographical Distribution of Board-Certified Physicians." *New England Journal of Medicine* 303(1980):1032–1038.

Seligman, M. *Helplessness: On Depression, Development, and Death.* San Francisco: W.H. Freeman & Company, 1975.

Severinghaus, A.E. "Distribution of Graduates of Medical Schools in the United States and Canada According to Specialties, 1900–1963." *Journal of Medical Education* 40(1965):721–736.

Shah, F.K., and Abbey, H. "Effects of Some Factors on Neonatal and Post-Neonatal Mortality, Analysis by Binary Variable Multiple Regression Method." *Milbank Memorial Fund Quarterly* 49(1969):33–57.

Sherwood, S. *Long-Term Care: A Handbook for Researchers, Planners, and Providers.* New York: Spectrum Publications, 1975.

Sherwood, S., and Feldman, C.S. "The Use of Easily Obtained Pre-coded Data in Screening Applicants to a Long-Term Care Facility." *Gerontologist* 10(1970):182–188.

Solon, J.A., and Greenawalt, L.F. "Physicians' Participation in Nursing Homes." *Medical Care* 12(1974):486–497.

Stevens, R. "Trends in Medical Specialization in the United States." *Inquiry* 8(1971):9–19.

Stout, R.W. "Hospital Care of the Elderly: General or Geriatric Medicine." *Age and Aging* 8(1979):137–140.

Tenney, J.B.; White, K.L.; and Williamson, J.W. "National Ambulatory Medical Care Survey: Background and Methodology; 1967–1972." *NCHSR Vital and Health Statistics,* Series 2, no. 61, DHEW Publication no. (HRA) 74-1335. Washington, D.C.: U.S. Government Printing Office, 1974.

Timmer, E.J., and Kovar, M.G. "Expenses for Hospital and Institutional Care During the Last Year of Life for Adults Who Died in 1964 or 1965, United States." *Vital and Health Statistics,* Series 22, no. 11, PHS Publication no. 1000. Washington, D.C.: U.S. Government Printing Office, 1971.

Trapnell, G.R. "The Rising Cost of Catastrophic Illness." Mimeographed report for the National Center for Health Services Research, December 1977.

U.S. Comptroller General. *The Well-Being of Older People in Cleveland, Ohio.* Publication no. (HRD) 77-70. Washington, D.C.: U.S. Government Printing Office, 1977.

————. *Entering a Nursing Home—Costly Implications for Medicaid and the Elderly.* Publication no. PAD-80-12. Washington, D.C.: U.S. Government Printing Office, 1979.

U.S. Department of Commerce, Bureau of the Census. *1970 Census of Population.* Washington, D.C.: U.S. Government Printing Office, 1973.

————. *Current Population Reports,* Series P-20, No. 323, Government Printing Office, Washington, D.C., 1977a.

————. *Current Population Reports,* Series P-25, no. 704. Washington, D.C.: U.S. Government Printing Office, 1977b.

————. *Current Population Reports,* Series P-60, no. 108. Washington, D.C.: Government Printing Office, 1977c.

————. *Social Indicators, 1976.* Washington, D.C.: U.S. Government Printing Office, 1977d.

U.S. Department of Health, Education and Welfare (DHEW). *Physicians for a Growing America: Report of the Surgeon General's Consultant Group on Medical Education* (The "Bane Report"). Washington, D.C.: U.S. Government Printing Office, 1959.

————. *Vital Statistics of the United States,* vol. 1. Washington, D.C.: U.S. Government Printing Office, 1970.

————. *Vital Statistics of the United States,* vol. 2. Washington, D.C.: U.S. Government Printing Office, 1973.

————. "Current Estimates from the Health Interview Study, United States." *Vital and Health Statistics,* Series 10, no. 119. Washington, D.C.: U.S. Government Printing Office, 1976.

————. *Working Document on Patient Care Management.* Washington, D.C.: U.S. Government Printing Office, 1978a.

————. *Long-Term Care Minimum Data Set.* Preliminary report of the

Technical Consultant Panel on the Long-Term Care Data Set, U.S. National Committee on Vital and Health Statistics. Washington, D.C.: U.S. Government Printing Office, 1978b.

————. *Health, United States, 1978.* Publication no. (PHS) 78-1232. Washington, D.C.: U.S. Government Printing Office, 1978c.

————. *Monthly Vital Statistics: Final Mortality Statistics, 1976,* vol. 26, no. 12. Washington, D.C.: U.S. Government Printing Office, 1978d.

U.S. Senate, Subcommittee on Long-Term Care of the Special Committee on Aging. *Nursing Home Care in the United States: Failure in Public Policy,* (Supporting Paper no. 3, *Doctors in Nursing Homes: The Shunned Responsibility*). Washington, D.C.: U.S. Government Printing Office, 1975.

University of Southern California, Division of Research in Medical Education (USC/DRME). *Psychiatry Practice Study Report, Medical Activities and Manpower Projects.* Los Angeles: USC School of Medicine, 1978.

Vincente, L.; Wiley, J.A.; and Carrington, R.A. "The Risk of Institutionalization Before Death." *Gerontologist* 19(1979):361-367.

Weissert, W.G. "Costs of Adult Day Care: A Comparison to Nursing Homes." *Inquiry* 15(1978):10-19.

Wilensky, H.L. *The Welfare State and Equality: Structural and Ideological Roots of Public Expenditures.* Los Angeles: University of California Press, 1975.

Willard, W. *Meeting the Challenge of Family Practice: Report of the AMA ad hoc Committee of Education for Family Practice.* Chicago: American Medical Association, 1966.

Willemain, T. *Patterns of Physician Visits to Nursing Home Patients,* University Health Policy Consortium Discussion Paper no. 19. Waltham, Mass.: Brandeis University, 1979.

Williams, T.F.; Hill, J.G.; Fairbank, M.E.; and Knox, K.G. "Appropriate Placement of the Chronically Ill and Aged." *Journal of the American Medical Association* 226(1973):1332-1335.

Williamson, J. "Notes on the Historical Development of Geriatric Medicine as a Medical Specialty." *Age and Ageing* 8(1979a):144-148.

————. "Geriatric Medicine: Whose Specialty?" *Annals of Internal Medicine* 91(1979b):774-777.

Wilson, R.W., and White, E.L. "Changes in Morbidity, Disability, and Utilization Differentials Between the Poor and the Nonpoor: Data from the Health Interview Survey, 1964 and 1973." *Medical Care* 15 (1977):636-646.

World Health Organization (WHO). *Training of Physicians for Family Practice.* Geneva: World Health Organization, 1963.

Index

AAGP. *See* American Academy of General Practice

AAMC. *See* Association of American Medical Colleges

ACEP. *See* American College of Emergency Physicians

AMA. *See* American Medical Association

Academic geriatricians, 41–42, 47–51, 93, 95–96

Academic geropsychiatrists, 64–65

ACCESS program (Rochester, N.Y.), 40, 100, 125

Administration on Aging, 32, 33, 94

Advisory Board of Medical Specialties, 81

"Aged," defined, 131

Aged poor, the, 12–13

Aged population: size and percentage of total population, 9–10

"Ageism" (Butler), 28, 83, 92

Aging cohorts, 126

Aiken, L.H., et al., 44, 72

Akpom, C.A., and S. Meyer, 30

Alameda County, Calif., 126

Ambulatory care, 20, 94

American Academy of Family Physicians, 18, 49

American Academy of General Practice, 81

American Academy of Pediatricians, 80

American Association for Geriatric Psychiatry, 67

American Association of Retired Persons, 30

American Board of Family Practice, 81

American Board of General Practice, 81

American Board of Medical Specialties, 81

American Board of Pediatricians, 80

American Board of Psychiatry and Neurology, 67

American College of Emergency Physicians, 18

American College of Physicians, 18

American College of Surgeons, 18

American Geriatrics Society, 1, 18, 83, 84

American Medical Association: *Annual Profile of Medical Practice* (1978), 17, 147; Council on Medical Education, 81; *Journal,* 80; Physician Survey (1977), 16–20, 67, 84, 92, 142, 148, 149, 150; Section Council for General Practice, 81

American Medical Student Association, 30–31, 32, 49–50

American Pediatrics Society, 80

American Psychiatrics Association, 18, 67

Anderson, W.F., 100

Arkansas College of Medicine, 30

Assessment function, 109–110

Association of American Medical Colleges, 30, 51

Battelle Health and Population Study Center, 33n, 147

Beard, Owen, 39

Binstock, R.H., 16

Binstock, R.H., and E. Shanas (eds.), 117

Birren, J.E., and K.W. Schaie (eds.), 117

Birren, J.E., and R.B. Sloane, 66, 67

Birth rate, 9

Blacks, 10, 12, 139, 140

Bloom, M., 102

Boston University, 68

Brocklehurst, J.C., et al., 40, 100

Bunker, J.P., 136

Burdick bill, 31–32

Butler, R., 16, 92

COSTEP. *See* Public Health Service:

About the Authors

Robert L. Kane, M.D., is professor of medicine in the Multi-Campus Division of Geriatric Medicine at the UCLA School of Medicine and professor of health services at the UCLA School of Public Health. He is also a senior researcher in the Health Sciences Program at The Rand Corporation. His work has covered a variety of topics related to health-services research and delivery of improved health care. Much of this research has been focused on long-term care. In collaboration with Rosalie A. Kane, he has published two other volumes on long-term care (*Long-Term Care in Six Countries* and *Assessing the Elderly: A Practical Guide to Measurement*). Dr. Kane serves as a consultant to a number of federal, state, and local agencies. He is the recipient of a National Institute on Aging Geriatric Medicine Academic Award. He is also the editor of *Journal of Community Health*.

David H. Solomon, M.D., is professor and executive chair of the Department of Medicine at UCLA School of Medicine. Among his many distinctions, Dr. Solomon is past president of the American Thyroid Association, current president of the Association of Professors of Medicine, and a member of the Institute of Medicine of the National Academy of Sciences. An endocrinologist with special expertise in thyroid disease, he has recently directed his attention to the problems of geriatric care in the United States. He spent his sabbatical year at The Rand Corporation working on policies related to the improvement of health care for the aged. This book is an outgrowth of a portion of that activity.

John C. Beck, M.D., is professor and director of the Multi-Campus Division of Geriatric Medicine at the UCLA School of Medicine. He was formerly chairman of the Department of Medicine at McGill University, director of the Robert Wood Johnson Foundation Clinical Scholar Program, and professor of medicine at University of California, San Francisco. A distinguished leader in American and international medicine, he is a former president of the American Board of Medical Specialties and a former chairman of the American Board of Internal Medicine. Dr. Beck is interested in the problems of medical education and the training of health personnel. He is now actively involved in developing geriatric programs as director of the UCLA/USC Long-Term Care Gerontology Center and chairman of the White House Conference on Aging's Technical Committee on Health Services. Dr. Beck spent his sabbatical year at The Rand Corporation working on care of the aged, which led to the material presented in this volume.

Emmett B. Keeler, Ph.D., is a mathematician for The Rand Corporation and a faculty member of Rand Graduate Institute. His recent book, *Cholesterol, Children, and Heart Disease: An Analysis of Alternatives* (with Berwick and Cretin), combines economics, mathematics, and epidemiology to evaluate a variety of programs. He has worked extensively in the Rand Health Insurance Study on the theory and estimation of the effects of copayment on medical care.

Rosalie A. Kane, D.S.W., is a researcher in the Health Sciences Program at The Rand Corporation and a part-time faculty member at UCLA School of Social Welfare. She is well known in the field of social work for her theory building and writings on subjects related to interprofessional teamwork, social-service delivery in health settings, and long-term care. Since August 1979 she has been editor-in-chief of *Health and Social Work,* a quarterly journal of the National Association of Social Workers. She was formerly an associate professor at University of Utah School of Social Work. Her Rand work has concentrated on long-term-care problems, and most recently she has been studying assessment measurements and techniques for clinical practice and research. She is coauthor, with Robert L. Kane, of a book on that subject, *Assessing the Elderly: A Practical Guide to Measurement* (Lexington Books, 1981).

Selected Rand Books

Armor, David J.; Polich, J. Michael; and Stambul, Harriet B. *Alcoholism and Treatment.* New York: John Wiley and Sons, 1978.

Brewer, Garry D., and Kakalik, James S. *Handicapped Children: Strategies for Improving Services.* New York: McGraw-Hill, 1979.

Bruno, James E., ed. *Emerging Issues in Education: Policy Implications for the Schools.* Lexington, Mass.: Lexington Books, D.C. Heath and Company, 1972.

Carpenter-Huffman, P., Kletter, R.C.; and Yin, R.K. *Cable Television— Developing Community Services.* New York: Crane, Russak and Company, 1975.

Comstock, George; Chaffee, Steven; Katzman, Natan; McCombs, Maxwell; and Roberts, Donald. *Television and Human Behavior.* New York: Columbia University Press, 1978.

Dalkey, Norman C. *Studies in the Quality of Life: Delphi and Decision-Making.* Lexington, Mass.: D.C. Heath and Company, 1972.

Greenwood, Peter W.; Chaiken, Jan M.; and Petersilia, Joan. *The Criminal Investigation Process.* Lexington, Mass.: Lexington Books, D.C. Heath and Company, 1977.

Kane, Rosalie A., and Kane, Robert L. *Assessing the Elderly: A Practical Guide to Measurement.* Lexington, Mass.: Lexington Books, D.C. Heath and Company, 1981.

Kane, Robert L.; Solomon, David, H.; Beck, John C.; and Kane, Rosalie A. *Geriatrics in the United States.* Lexington, Mass.: Lexington Books, D.C. Heath and Company, 1981.

McLaughlin, Milbrey Wallin. *Evaluation and Reform: The Elementary and Secondary Education Act of 1965/Title I.* Cambridge, Mass.: Ballinger Publishing Company, 1975.

Park, Rolla Edward. *The Role of Analysis in Regulatory Decisionmaking.* Lexington, Mass.: D.C. Heath and Company, 1973.

Quade, E.S. *Analysis for Public Decisions.* New York: American Elsevier Publishing Company, 1975.

Sackman, Harold. *Delphi Critique: Expert Opinion, Forecasting, and Group Process.* Lexington, Mass.: D.C. Heath and Company, 1975.

Smith, James P. *Female Labor Supply.* Princeton, N.J.: Princeton University Press, 1980.

Timpane, Michael, ed. *The Federal Interest in Financing Schooling.* Cambridge, Mass.: Ballinger Publishing Company, 1978.

Wirt, John G.; Lieberman, Arnold J.; and Levien, Roger E. *R&D Management: Methods Used by Federal Agencies.* Lexington, Mass.: D.C. Heath and Company, 1975.

Yin, Robert K.; Bateman, Peter M.; Marks, Ellen L. and Quick, Suzanne K. *Changing Urban Bureaucracies: How New Practices Get Routinized.* Lexington, Mass.: Lexington Books, D.C. Heath and Company, 1979.
Yin, Robert K., and Yates, Douglas. *Street-Level Governments: Assessing Decentralization and Urban Systems.* Lexington, Mass.: Lexington Books, D.C. Heath and Company, 1975.